Cancer
with
JOY

How to Transform Fear

into HAPPINESS

and Find the Bright Side Effects

Joy Huber

foreword by Susie Huber

NEW YORK

Cancer with JOY

How to Transform Fear into Happiness and Find the Bright Side Effects

by **Joy Huber**

ISBN 978-1-61448-101-0 Paperback
ISBN 978-1-61448-102-7 ePub Version
Library of Congress Control Number: 2011935310

Published by:
MORGAN JAMES PUBLISHING
The Entrepreneurial Publisher
5 Penn Plaza, 23rd Floor
New York City, New York 10001
(212) 655-5470 Office
(516) 908-4496 Fax
www.MorganJamesPublishing.com

Editing by:
Hallagen Ink

Cover Design by:
Rachel Lopez
rachel@r2cdesign.com

Interior Design by:
Bonnie Bushman
bbushman@bresnan.net

To buy books in quantity, call 402-560-1861 or e-mail books@cancerwithjoy.com.

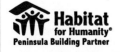

In an effort to support local communities, raise awareness and funds, Morgan James Publishing donates one percent of all book sales for the life of each book to Habitat for Humanity.

Get involved today, visit
www.HelpHabitatForHumanity.org.

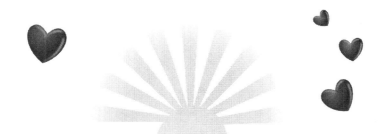

Dedication

This book is dedicated, first and foremost, to all those who use it. Whether you are a newly diagnosed cancer patient, a caregiver, or someone else playing an integral role on the support team like a family member or friend, there is so much valuable time, energy, and money-saving information in here to be utilized. I have no doubt this resource can help you face "Cancer with Joy"—when used.

Secondly, I dedicate this to my family, including my maternal Grandpa Kreifel who passed two months after my diagnosis on Tuesday, May 25, 2010. Thank You for showing so much more through your example and also by your words. A Special Thank You to my mom Susie Huber (my primary caregiver during cancer treatment) for her constant love and for being there for me no matter what! When I look back over this entire life journey, you have been in my corner no matter what I was tackling, from stage four cancer to writing a book!

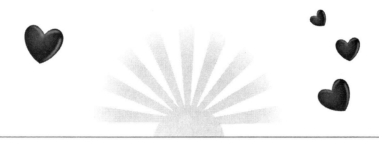

Acknowledgements

I want to acknowledge so many for their assistance in making this all happen. First, a very heartfelt sincere Thank You goes to everyone at my wonderful publisher, Morgan James Publishing, who worked on "Cancer with Joy" as we transformed a tremendous idea to really helping the newly diagnosed and everyone on their support team. I have been so honored to work with all of you and look forward to a lifelong relationship. Rick Frishman, asking for my book proposal truly changed my life! I cannot Thank You enough for the brilliant ideas you contributed. Special Thanks also to David, Margo, Bethany, Jim, and Cindy. Thank You Tanya at Hallagen Ink for your help editing my draft into this beautiful resource.

Thank You also to my eleven contributors for sharing their personal stories in chapter three.

Jan Hasak	Edward Leigh, M.A.
Steve Hilgenfeld	Cristy Norwood
Lois Tschetter Hjelmstad	Anna Renault
Elaine Jesmer	Marie Rowe
Diana Kaaha	Hayley Townley
Gail King	

*Thank You to <u>all</u> those I cite throughout the book who allowed me to share their work with you as part of "Cancer with Joy." Thank You Rachel Pappas, Author of "Hopping Roller Coasters," <u>www.1uponcancer. com</u>; Larry Camerlin, Air Charity Network; Sharon Blynn, Bald Is Beautiful, <u>www.baldisbeautiful.org</u>; Dennis W. Pyritz, Being Cancer Network, <u>www.beingcancer.net</u>; Camp Kesem National; CANCER101 Inc.; Darryl Mitteldorf, LCSW, and the CancerMatch.com team; Cancer Support Community; Caregivers4Cancer; Circus of Cancer; Cooking With Cancer, Inc. "Prescription to Taste: A Cooking Guide For Cancer Patients"; Reprinted with Permission of Empowher.com; FamilyCare America, Inc.; FirstGiving Inc.; Kelly Malin, First Descents; GiveForward; Ginger Johnson, founder of HappyChemo.com and BoobsAreOptional.com; Hope Flight Foundation; Patty Murray, Hope for Two…The Pregnant with CANCER Network; Imerman Angels; I'm Too Young For This! Cancer Foundation; LIVE**STRONG**, <u>www.livestrong.org</u>; Lotsa Helping Hands; Margerie McNeill Manning; Musicians On Call; National Cervical Cancer Coalition (NCCC); OMNI Health Media; Christine B. Ferdinand, Operation Bling Foundation; Patient Advocate Foundation; Courtesy of The Personal Care Products Council Foundation c/o Look Good…Feel Better; "tlc" Catalog; U.S. News & World Report's 2010 ranking of Best Hospitals; Vital Options Int.; Wings of Angels; and YoungCancerSpouses.*

If I accidentally left anyone out, I sincerely apologize. I greatly appreciate your contribution to this important project.

Foreword

I have known Joy longer than anyone else, but I still felt honored when she asked me to write the foreword for her second book, *Cancer with Joy: How to Transform Fear into Happiness and Find the Bright Side Effects.* We went to the hospital in July of 1976 with several names in mind, but the first time they placed her in my arms I just knew she was "a bundle of joy," and we named her so! She was always a happy baby and a happy person in general.

Having lived longer, I think I have known more people who have faced a cancer diagnosis than Joy did since she was just thirty-three, and I know from experience that most have *not* handled "Cancer with Joy!" I have definitely watched Joy face many obstacles throughout her young life, but obviously none as life threatening or serious as this. A cancer diagnosis is devastating enough, let alone having it come as a young adult. I felt Joy was just beginning to really live her life; she had never married or had children. She was just several years into owning her own business and was still working very hard as an entrepreneur to build things up, as one must do in the beginning years.

As the pieces of the puzzle fell into place, we found out we were facing not only cancer, but stage four cancer with involvement in a major organ (the right kidney) as well as in the bone marrow. My heart was truly broken in pieces for my youngest child. She consistently lived true to her name of Joy, responding positively to life's challenges, but cancer was a completely different animal. Would this be the one thing that would break her spirit? I would not have blamed her for becoming angry, sad, and/or depressed amongst exhibiting other emotions.

I was not only proud but also pleased to watch her respond with humor and a positive attitude. Here she was handling a stage four cancer diagnosis as a young adult "with joy!" I think I as well as others around me responded in kind to how Joy was handling everything. We soon truly made the best of every challenging situation, including me getting into costume for trips to the hospital and surgery center around the holidays! Check out the generous bonus Joy included with your purchase of this book for pictures! If only others could hear her inspiring story, and learn how to handle something as devastating as "Cancer with Joy." I know it can be done. I watched first-hand.

When Joy had the idea for "Cancer with Joy," I thought it was absolutely phenomenal, but was convinced surely someone somewhere in the entire world would already be doing this to give to and help others. Surely my daughter was not the first person named Joy who was diagnosed with stage four cancer, handling it well, and already out there teaching others. We checked the domain www.cancerwithjoy.com to see what was there and what was being done to help others further back on the road from diagnosis through treatment. Nothing was there! I was truly shocked but felt this was the Lord's mission for my daughter to give back to and help millions of others.

And so a "Cancer with Joy" logo was created, it was filed with the United States Patent and Trademark Office, and you hold in your hands the essential resource that can transform your fear and experience into… "Cancer with Joy."

—Susie Huber

Table of Contents

Chapter One

The "Cancer with Joy" Story

We do not know with certainty when we awake what each day will reveal to us. We can make plans, but "life happens." Many days are uneventful, meaning we do things but of no significance and have no strong memories from those days. On other days, big events and life changing things happen over those twenty-four hours, and we will forever remember the day going forward.

Birthdays are days most people enjoy remembering and celebrating each year. Some people say, "Oh, it is just another day." Well, I will *never* feel that way about another birthday. Not after the events that took place between my thirty-third and thirty-fourth birthdays!

In my thirty-four quick years on this earth, I do not recall anything particularly special about "March 12." It does not stand out for me as a day I should remember like a friend's birthday, etc. Well, that all changed Friday, March 12, 2010.

Events in my life had almost lined up perfectly. I should have known a major curveball was ahead! I had *finally* decided you have to **do** things you want to do instead of sitting back and wondering, "What if?" Go for it and then you will *know*!

I was born in a very small town in Southeast Nebraska in 1976 and have <u>always</u> lived within a three-hour radius of there. I went to one school K–12 so the idea of moving is a big deal for me. I started songwriting as a hobby in late 2005, after the unexpected passing of my paternal grandma.

The year of 2005 is one that stands out for me as a "big year" full of life altering events and dates! I lost my second grandparent, but it was my first passing since I had been "an adult" and I could comprehend a big loss of family this close to me. The best paying job I had ever held was "eliminated" while I was a single homeowner. *And* I decided to tap my entrepreneurial spirit and start my own business in public speaking and training (www.JoyHuber.com).

As my involvement with my songwriting hobby deepened, I began seriously contemplating making the move from Lincoln, Nebraska, where my home was, to Nashville, Tennessee. "Why not? WHAT was holding me back?" I had to ask. I was single, never married in fact, with no children to uproot, and I had my own business that could be based anywhere. As long as I was close to a major airport where I could fly in and out to travel to speaking engagements, I had satisfied the major requirement for my business.

My last serious boyfriend and relationship happened in 2007, and when I broke up with him, I promised myself not to let *a man* and a relationship break my momentum in building my business and going for my dreams again! I was spending so much time with him at his request instead of putting in the necessary non-paid time to build a business (blogging, tweeting, marketing, etc.). When the relationship ended up not working out, I was regretful.

Bound and determined not to make that mistake again, I hired a professional coach in 2008 and got down to doing the hard work or putting in "sweat equity" I think it is called. I remained single by choice and kept my focus on my new, clearly defined work mission. By late 2009, I had made progress and felt ready for a move. I do not know exactly what constitutes ready; it is surely different for each person. I can say that when you are ready, you know it, and I was there!

Around Christmas 2009, I announced to my parents my intent of listing my home by early spring, selling, and hopefully being in Nashville in time to enjoy the cool, crisp fall weather. I could tell they were saddened by my decision to move so far away from home, as my only other sibling lives, you guessed it, within driving distance! I could also tell they knew my resolve and there was no changing my mind. The best option was to show support for this "thing" that was happening in 2010 or be alienated in the process of opposing it.

Valentine's Day of 2010 found me not out with a date, but going through things in the spare bedroom where all the stuff accumulated to clear the clutter. No sense paying to move all this stuff to Tennessee and *then* go through it and toss it out there! I intended to list my house March 1, and ran a day behind getting it on the market March 2. Here come all those life changing dates I will never forget!

Tuesday, March 9, 2010: "R u in Lincoln?" This short text comes in from an ex-boyfriend (but Facebook friend) while I was at my parents with all my tax items spread out on their living room floor. I was putting my 2009 business and personal records together for my accountant. I respond that I am not, but he must be, otherwise why would he inquire if *I* were in the city. I find out he is in town with his job for the week staying at the Downtown Holiday Inn. Basically, would I want to meet for a drink?

Interesting. I met him on my twenty-first birthday in 1997, and we had dated off and on a few times throughout the years, most recently in

August 2008. I stayed friends with him and was always intrigued at how much he was "just like me" meaning he too had never married or had kids. Those are big pluses for me in a life partner; since I have not been through these big experiences, ideally they have not either.

Wednesday, March 10, 2010: My house amazingly sold in record time—I should have asked for more—eight days with only one Sunday Open House. I was back in Lincoln that morning to sign papers, have lunch with a dear friend to celebrate her birthday (a significant date), work with a coaching client via phone (I am professionally trained in coaching and *love* working with people individually), and then, yes, meet the ex-boyfriend at the Downtown Holiday Inn bar for that drink and conversation. There were others at the bar and there was a bunch of joking around, which was fun, but it did not allow me to tell him of my Tennessee future. He deserved to be clued in. We went up to his room to talk (sincerely, just talk), and we received much teasing from the bar group when we disappeared.

I informed him of my house selling, and gave him my timeline for Tennessee. I was going out there in two weeks for an event with the Songwriters Association and attending the "Tin Pan South" music festival in early April. I was also working with a Realtor out there to line up my future living arrangements. I told him when my house would close, and when my parents and I intended to load a truck with my furniture and drive to Tennessee. After unloading, I would begin my new exciting life. He got the most faraway look in his eyes I have ever seen, said, "Huh," and not much else!

I felt rather sad that night too because I still felt a connection to him and could not help but wonder, "What if we had tried just *one* more time?" He really seemed to have matured since the August 2008 time we had spent together. But I was resolved that Tennessee time had *finally* come and **nothing** was stopping me. No *person* certainly.

Friday, March 12, 2010: My concerned mom had previously noticed some lumps on my neck. She had pushed on them, asked me if they hurt, to which I responded, "Nope, no problems there." Seeing my imminent move east, she scheduled an appointment for me with a doctor "just to make sure." I remember telling her it would be a waste of my money on an office call fee since I was uninsured as a small business owner. Sometimes we are so wrong but just do not know it yet.

The doctor felt around my neck, asked me the customary questions like if the multiple lumps hurt, how long I had noticed them, etc., and said a lot of one word I remember: "Hmmm…."

He ended up ordering a CT (computerized tomography) scan and before I knew it I was being taken in for an IV (intravenous), which is one of my least favorite things in the world. To make matters worse, the nurse hit a vein valve in the first hand she tried, and had to bandage it up. "Give me your other hand," she said.

"You're kidding me," I said, trying to use humor as I do to handle challenging situations. "Okay, but after this I am out of hands so I hope we get it this time." We both laughed!

A stat read was ordered on the CT scan, and when we saw my doctor again, what he said exactly gets fuzzy for me. My mind took off thinking so many other things. I was trying to listen to what he said, but definitely did not get it all. Something about best case scenario I had a bad infection, and he would prescribe an antibiotic two times a day for seven days to see if he could clear that up. Worst case scenario though I remember him saying, "Lymphoma."

I remember saying, ***"Can-cer???"*** He explained he would set me up to see an ENT (Ear, Nose, and Throat doctor) the next week.

Not to get out of order here, but did I mention Friday, March 26, 2010? That was a date I had **plans**. I had a flight scheduled into Nashville, rental car booked to pick-up, and friends I was planning to stay with. Suddenly my "plans" and perfect timeline were very questionable.

Thursday, March 18, 2010: I met with an ENT that there was NO WAY I was going to work with due to his extreme lack of bedside manner and poor communication with patient and family. Whether you are reading this due to your diagnosis, or as the caregiver, family, or friend to someone newly diagnosed, remember it is YOUR health and you have the right to work with a doctor who makes you comfortable. We ended up going "around" this guy! His nurse scheduled me for an ultrasound needle biopsy to needle into the enlarged lymph nodes and pull out cells for testing.

In the meantime, my house passed its inspection and a "SOLD" sign went over the "For Sale" sign in the yard. Days that should have been so happy for me because my dream of moving away to Nashville to answer the "What if?" became muddled with online searches about "lymphoma" to quickly educate myself. There were also many vague Facebook postings because I needed to let true friends know "something" was up, but then there are all the Facebook "friends" from back home you are not *really* friends with you know, and I did not need the small-town rumor mill churning, "Did you hear about Joy Huber? Yeah, she's got cancer!" Nothing had been confirmed yet, but having the word mentioned was bad enough.

Friday, March 19, 2010: I had an early-morning appointment at the hospital for the ultrasound needle biopsy. As the deadening wore off, I felt some pretty intense pain coupled with the anxiety of not having anything confirmed, so I cancelled plans to be at a group dinner with dear friends and former co-workers that evening. I had even planned to host the after-dinner drinks at my house, have everyone pull up and see the "SOLD" sign I thought I would be so proud of, and reveal my big plans. Those plans faded with uncertainty over my health. In the days following, before anything was confirmed, I about went bananas. But ....

Wednesday, March 24, 2010 (I also call this "D-Day" for "Diagnosis Day"): Just two short weeks after signing papers on my house, seeing the ex to share my big plans, and having my first doctor's appointment where he was so concerned about those lumps in my neck, I received confirmation that I had indeed, "Lymphoma CANCER." **NOT at thirty-three?!** I remember standing in my bathroom, looking in the mirror at my reflection, saying, "You have cancer. YOU have cancer. YOU HAVE CAN-CER." I still could not completely wrap my mind around it. Yes, I could see the lumps in my neck, and I could feel the tumors too, but I FELT fine.

Surely there was a mix-up with my results and someone else was supposed to be hearing the news they were accidentally delivering to me. I mean, I've seen *Last Holiday* with Queen Latifah, and she was misdiagnosed (Paramount Pictures 1996). Surely the same thing would be revealed to me. SURELY. Yet DATES continued to fill with appointments now.

Friday, March 26, 2010: Remember I had said this was the day I was to fly away to Nashville? This was now the day I had a PET (positron-emission tomography) scan, and my first appointment with my oncologist.

The next week, I had a medical appointment *every single day*. I have found that having stage four Non-Hodgkin's Follicular Lymphoma often feels like a full-time job between trying to educate yourself to be an empowered patient, and going to all these appointments. No one will DO anything for you without seeing you first, so there are many "Initial Consultations." Ugh! The week of March 29th when I was supposed to be looking at living arrangements by day and hearing fabulous live music by night at the Bluebird Café and other terrific Nashville venues became:

Monday—"Initial Consultation" with *new* (and *much* improved) ENT.

Tuesday—"Initial Consultation" with a urologist. (I am a little embarrassed to have had one of those at my age. At the doctor's office, most of the people in the waiting room were my grandparents' age.) One of my tests revealed a swollen lymph node almost sealing off the ureter, an important tube that drains urine from your kidneys to your bladder. While a little gross, if we cannot remove our wastes from our bodies, it becomes a toxic situation very quickly. This was the case for me.

I had to have a stent put in place from the bladder up the ureter into the right kidney to keep the ureter open so that kidney could drain. My oncologist made it clear that this was "VERY important" that it happen, like, yesterday. I understood his sense of urgency and, unfortunately, so did my concerned mom I described earlier. (Did I mention I am the youngest, and unmarried, so she was my primary "caregiver?")

Wednesday—Physical to get cleared for procedures being scheduled to occur that same week due to urgency.

Thursday—In hospital to have incision in neck to remove big bulging lymph node to determine the type of lymphoma. (Ironically, *this* was April Fools' Day!)

Friday—Back to hospital to have anesthesia including breathing tube before another surgery to place the stent in my right kidney. (When the doctor was worried about my kidney not being able to drain and thus shutting down, I said to it many times in an encouraging tone, "Hang in there kidneys! Help is on the way!" I would laugh at this, but saying it aloud helped to also remind me that help *was* on the way now that I had been diagnosed.)

There are many more dates that stick out here as a new cancer diagnosis puts you on quite a path of *frequent* interaction with medical professionals. I had to have a bone marrow aspiration to have marrow tested, and yes, the cancer was in the bone marrow too. I have often wondered how this could spread and spread and I had no idea and felt healthy. I do not obsess about it though; questions like that will drive you bananas!

I chose to have a port placed in my upper left chest to deliver the chemotherapy (chemo). It was either that or I would have frequent IVs. You read earlier those are about my least favorite thing in the world! Chemotherapy is what was prescribed for my initial treatment as we gained a complete picture from all the tests.

In the meantime, I am so proud to say I took off driving to Arkansas (with Mom in tow, no way was she letting me go alone!) for I had a confirmed contract speaking engagement with Arkansas Phi Beta Lambda (college division of Future Business Leaders of America, and I am a proud PBL Alum!). I had bone marrow taken out for testing in Lincoln, Nebraska on April 7; did my speaking engagement in Little Rock, Arkansas on Friday morning, April 9; had the chemo port placed after returning to Lincoln, Nebraska on Monday, April 12; and had my first chemo treatment on Wednesday, April 14! It was three weeks to the day after my diagnosis.

"They" (my oncologist, and a top lymphoma specialist from the University of Nebraska Medical Center in Omaha, Nebraska) prescribed six rounds of five different chemo medicines. Each of the six rounds was delivered three weeks apart. So that let me know what to expect for the next five months.

Cancer is a long road I do not think anyone ever plans or believes *they* will go down, but too many of us get detoured onto it in the midst of "living life" or even "getting by." I fought like crazy to "look normal" and look the same, but I also wanted desperately to be acknowledged for that fight. Some people feel since I look "fine," I am "just fine," and my huge courageous battle is "nothing." They dismiss it, which has been very disappointing and frustrating for me.

Cancer is war raging *inside* your body, and with that huge internal battle going on, you will have external side effects. Losing my hair was definitely the most emotionally painful thing that happened. I had shoulder-length hair at diagnosis. (See the end of this book for a bonus telling you about a companion website to visit to see many pictures and video from my journey!) At my first chemo, they informed me I had approximately two-to-three weeks before it would start coming out. I *really* did not want chunks of hair that long coming out.

I decided to take control of as much of this as I could versus letting things happen, and I cut my hair very short the same day I closed on my house: Thursday, April 22, 2010. It still was coming out on my pillow. After taking one shower where I honestly believed I would have no hair left—I saw what came out in my hands when I shampooed and heard and saw what hit the drain as I rinsed—I decided to shave my head. Since hair loss was the most emotionally painful part of my cancer experience, I will talk about this more in other chapters in the book. In the next chapter, I will even tell you how I took the *most* emotionally painful moment and handled it with joy!

After six intense chemo treatments (one in April, two in May, one in June, one in July, and one in August) I achieved remission in September 2010! But my treatment story does not end there. My doctors prescribed TWELVE additional rounds of "maintenance chemo," now occurring every eight weeks apart. I am reminded that cancer treatment is a marathon, not a sprint! As of writing this book in the spring of 2011, I have had four of the twelve maintenance chemo treatments, and—best case scenario—have eight more to go!

Regarding the port that was implanted in April 2010, I recently celebrated its one-year birthday because, the way my doctor's said it to me, "We will have our next Presidential Election in November of 2012 before that port comes out. Make friends with it." It has been with me a year now and it will be with me another eighteen months!

Since I have achieved remission, the whole idea of "Cancer with Joy" overpowered me and I knew it was my life's mission and purpose! It was just too interesting with the double meaning since thankfully I was named Joy. For you, it means handling "Cancer with Joy," literally, with me in your corner. I am here for you throughout your experience as a valuable resource. It also means I will inspire you and show you how to face "Cancer with Joy," figuratively, by sharing examples of how I did it even with a stage four cancer diagnosis as a young adult. I believe strongly in using the power of positivity, the power of a positive attitude, and humor to respond to whatever obstacles life throws our way.

In his book *The Success Principles* (2005), author Jack Canfield writes, "E + R = O (Event + Response = Outcome)." He later states, "You can instead simply change your responses (R) to the events (E)— the way things are—until you get the outcomes (O) you want." This is why people can experience the same event, but produce different results. Their individual response to that event is what makes all the difference. Canfield also says, "You only have control over three things in your life— the thoughts you think, the images you visualize, and the actions you take (your behavior)."

I knew of this formula, fortunately, long before my cancer diagnosis and have made a conscious effort to apply these principles to my life both professionally and personally. To me, it is so significant that E does not equal O. *This* event does not automatically dictate *this* outcome. You get to factor in your response, or shall I say, how you *choose* to respond, and that is what ultimately dictates the outcome.

Being diagnosed with cancer (certainly a big event) does not mean the outcome is automatically (pick one or all): you are angry, bitter, depressed, and/or sad! You can and will control, as Canfield says, the thoughts you think and the actions you take.

I certainly have my critics of the idea of "Cancer with Joy." I was so thrilled with the idea I had a logo designed with the sun actually rising out of the word cancer! How dare I, you might ask? To me, that warm yellow sun rising out of this c-word suggests hope, warmth, optimism, even the gratitude that comes from each new day and the opportunity we have to live and to fight. The red hearts in the logo drifting upwards signify love and compassion. I have all of these feelings regularly and I have all of them for you, too, as you begin and continue your cancer experience.

I have had such a favorable response to the logo and putting this new idea out there about facing "Cancer with Joy" using positivity instead of negativity, that I have been overwhelmed by requests for this logo on products including T-shirts. Many Christian women's groups in particular have been interested in products that acknowledge, "Yes, I (or someone I love and support!) have this going on, but we are fighting it using positivity." I have seen other T-shirts that have negativity or even profanity on them with the word cancer and knew there was plenty of room for "Cancer with Joy" out there too!

The basic premise behind "Cancer with Joy" is we realize no one is happy they have cancer, BUT you can have cancer and still be happy. WOW, what an insight! Hopefully you will agree and make the decision that even though you or someone you love has cancer, you can still be happy. You can choose to respond to it with joy! Remember I am in your corner and here for you each step of the way. The bonus at the back of the book will explain how you can stay connected to me way beyond just reading this resource.

There is one final thing I will say about this, regarding people who have said, "Easy for you to say. Did a doctor ever tell *you*, 'You have three months; make the most of it'?"

No, I never heard that. I worked with a doctor who made me feel like, "This *is* very serious (there is no stage five cancer after all!), but there is a lot we can do to fix it, fight it, etc."

While I wondered at diagnosis and definitely braced (and tried to prepare) myself to hear words like that giving me a marked time period in which I had to live, I did not hear that. People ask, "If you *had* heard you only had three months, or three weeks, to live, do you *really* think you would still be handling 'Cancer with Joy?'"

The answer, without a doubt, is yes! Especially then. Even more so then! If I found out my cancer was terminal and I had a very limited amount of time to live, I would wholeheartedly propose handling it with joy because time is really of the essence then. Do you really want to spend your last few years, months, weeks, days, whatever time you have, left on earth in a bad mood, angry, bitter, depressed, and/or sad?

I understand the crying; I am not going to try to tell you I never cried over my diagnosis. You should not misunderstand "Cancer with Joy" as me saying you should *always* be happy and *not* cry over your diagnosis. Remember I said at "Cancer with Joy" we realize no one is happy they have cancer! In chapter four, I will share a dozen things you need to know of recommended dos and don'ts at diagnosis.

I believe, especially when "bad" or challenging things happen to all of us in life, we are tempted to ask, "Why?" "Why me?" I personally never found myself obsessing about "Why me?" and why this happened to me. Instead I have felt, "Why not me?" Lots of people have to face a cancer diagnosis every single day. ("About 3,400 people are diagnosed with cancer each day in the U.S.," according to http://cancer.about.com/od/cancerfactsandstatistics/f/dailydeaths.htm.) So why not *me*? I found that question coming to me over and over again. I am probably a lot like you; there is nothing that special about me that says I should be exempt from cancer for my whole life. Cancer certainly does not discriminate; it impacts everyday people like me, celebrities, rich, poor, men, women, the elderly, children, and even babies, unfortunately!

Perhaps because I knew of the E + R = O formula, I said, "This cancer event is happening, but I *know* it is my response to this that will ultimately dictate the outcome." I have chosen to focus on what positive things I can do with my diagnosis instead of letting it happen to me and not finding good that *can* come of it. Before I was even diagnosed, I co-wrote a song called "Live Before I Die," about squeezing the most juice out of life.

After my diagnosis, it became one of my personal theme songs, more endeared to me than other songs out there since I co-wrote it. You can listen to it when you access the bonus at the end of this book! It could definitely be compared to the epic country song recorded by Tim McGraw "Live Like You Were Dying," but there are some important differences. Since I am a woman, this song has a woman's voice. Also, no one is presented as dying in the song like the character Tim McGraw is speaking to. "I wanna see how far I can go, when I put my heart in drive!" my co-writer and I wrote. What happens when you put *your* heart in drive and go, even with a cancer diagnosis present in your life?

In the next chapter, I want to share with you very specific examples of ways, ten ways, that I handled my cancer experience with joy! It is my sincere hope that these real examples of how I handled cancer with positivity, before the "Cancer with Joy" idea came to me, will inspire you to do the same. Then you can share your story of how you handled "Cancer with Joy" with me, and also help many others.

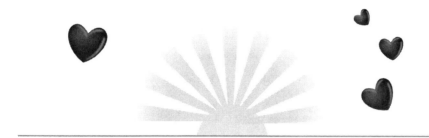

Chapter Two

Ten Ways to Handle "Cancer with Joy"

I know there are infinitely more than just ten ways to handle "Cancer with Joy." I have many more than ten from my experience so far. Remember as of this writing, I am still in maintenance chemotherapy. I continue to find new ways to handle "Cancer with Joy." I share these and additional funny stories in my live "Cancer with Joy" program you can read about at www.JoyHuber.com/programs. To book me as a speaker, simply complete the form at www.JoyHuber.com/contact.

In the next chapter, I will share some phenomenal stories from others I have learned about while writing. There is a wonderful book I would recommend to you called *Chicken Soup for the Soul: The Cancer Book (101 Stories of Courage, Support & Love)* by Jack Canfield, Mark Victor Hansen, and David Tabatsky (Chicken Soup for the Soul Publishing, LLC, 2009). You can get a copy at www.CancerwithJoy.com (right side of page). I certainly did not want to even attempt to do what was already done so well in that book. So when I looked for stories to put in this book, I only asked contributors to expound with specific examples on how *they* handled "Cancer with Joy." I *love* the stories that came in. I hope and believe you will too!

For space reasons here, I will share ten of my own personal examples of how I handled "Cancer with Joy." You can contribute your examples to stories@cancerwithjoybook.com for the opportunity to be featured online at the bonus website provided as a valuable add-on to this book. You could even be featured in a future book of mine!

Number One—Handle "Cancer with Joy" (even at the holidays!)

Here is my personal example. The very first holiday that occurred after my Wednesday, March 24, 2010 diagnosis was Easter. In 2010, Easter was on Sunday, April 4. This was the weekend after the first full week following my diagnosis, and I had a medical appointment or surgery scheduled *every single day that week* as noted in the previous chapter. In the days right before Easter, I had two surgeries scheduled to remove a lymph node from the right side of my neck (I mentioned earlier that this surgery ironically occurred on April Fools' Day) and to place a stent from my bladder into the right kidney on Good Friday, Friday, April 2, 2010.

I grew up with parents who had Mickey & Minnie Mouse costumes made to wear to a costume party in southeast Nebraska when I was in high school. I distinctly remember borrowing my mom's Minnie Mouse costume and wearing it out with friends on Halloween in high school and in college. Our family's philosophy has always been to make fun out of what we possibly can and not take life too seriously or go through it too stiffly!

My mom also had a complete Easter bunny costume with white furry zip-up suit (with bushy little tail), pull on white/pink paws, and of course, white/pink big ears! She asked and I encouraged her to wear this as my escort to the hospital for both surgical procedures on April Fools' Day *AND* on Good Friday.

Since three days after my diagnosis, I have had a free *CaringBridge* website to keep the masses of family and friends informed, saving considerable time and energy from trying to share the same information over and over. I will share more about CaringBridge in the last chapter, "Resources You Need to Know About (at Diagnosis)." Here is an excerpt from my CaringBridge journal posting Saturday, April 3, 2010.

> Since it's Easter weekend my mom has an Easter bunny costume complete with white furry zip-up suit, bunny ears, mitten paws, etc. All of you who know her will not be surprised to read this! We decided through all the tears being shed that laughter & humor is the best approach so I encouraged her to wear the bunny costume to the hospital!! ☺ She wore it Thurs. & Fri. and happily went to other rooms, as requested by hospital staff, to entertain children in the hospital for surgeries, etc. She really delighted them!

Not only were we handling "Cancer with Joy" and laughter, but we were helping others in the hospital for surgeries on my floor providing smiles and laughs for them too!

You should have seen the hospital staff—most focused on doing their jobs, but very serious and sober—when I walked up to check in for surgery with the Easter bunny in tow! It truly is how you respond that matters!

As part of the same example of handling "Cancer with Joy" at the holidays, after I achieved remission in September of 2010, I had an abnormal Pap smear escalate into cervical biopsies and the need for the LEEP (loop electrosurgical excision procedure) on Monday, December 13, 2010. With less than two weeks to go until Christmas, and surgical procedures <u>still</u> happening, Mom came with me to the surgery center with flashing reindeer antlers on her head! We definitely transformed many sober faces into laughter that day!

I said in my December 16 CaringBridge post:

> Mom said since this is STILL going on for me by Christmas time she would keep the spirit of dressing in costume & wear reindeer antlers. We were going to call her 'Rudolph,' but she didn't have the red nose. We settled on 'Prancer,' or 'Dancer.' Ha! We definitely like to cope with all this heavy medical stuff happening at a young age by having fun! We all have a **choice** in how we respond to life's challenges as I'm reminded of regularly!

Number Two—Name the cancer and joke about it!

When I found out I had lymphoma and it was these enlarged lymph nodes all over causing all these problems (threatening to shut my right kidney down), I decided to name the cancer. It was a real part of my life so I might as well acknowledge it. Now, there's no way I'm going to give it a "nice" name. I decided to name mine "Dick." When I tell this story live, it causes lots of giggles. I cracked jokes including that I had to pay rent or pay a mortgage in order to keep living in my house, and "Dick" was not paying rent to be living in my body. So, he would be forcibly removed with the help of the doctors, chemo medicines, prayers, and a positive attitude!

When I had surgery to remove "Dick" from my neck, I found ways to laugh that very night, saying all the cancer cells in my body were grouping up for dinner, and they said, "Guys? Um, GUYS! Has anyone seen Dick? Uh-oh! He's missing! Uh, do you think she knows about us being here rent-free? Is she onto us? Dick? I think she's going to remove us if we don't leave on our own."

I know that sounds like the silliest thing, but you do what works for you. That worked well for me, and brought me lots of comfort to think that the cancer cells trying to grow and spread further in my body were now running scared knowing they had been detected! When I have shared that story, many have appreciated and loved it! Others have said they were going to name their cancer too!

Number Three—Appreciation.

Another way I personally handled "Cancer with Joy" was by **gaining a new appreciation of, and joy for, the littlest things in life we all take for granted** but that brought me happiness. Even though I had stage four cancer, I still had and felt joy for so many people and things that made me happy.

I began my April 6, 2010 CaringBridge journal entry with the following:

> Good Evening, my companions as I write tonight's journal entry are Oreos (Double Stuff, mmm!) & a big mug of milk. We all forget to delight in the tiny things in life & that's one thing my diagnosis has given me. Delight & gratitude for things one might consider "small." Such as these yummy chocolate cookies! ☺

Then my mom's youngest sister sent me a package of Oreos in the mail!

The littlest things are often what mean the most! She read what sheer delight I was getting and thought to put a package in the mail. If you are reading this as a caregiver, friend, etc., of someone newly diagnosed, please remember it is not about big gestures, but the littlest (and thankfully, inexpensive) things that say, "I thought of you today!"

Number Four—Handling "Cancer with Joy" even at cancer treatment!

At my first chemo I quickly figured out this pole where the bags of my medicines hung was attached to me for the duration. I certainly was not used to something like that. Of course with all the liquid going in, I quickly had to use the restroom. After unplugging everything, I told the nurse "Jane and I are going to the bathroom. We'll be right back."

She looked at me and smiled. I said, "You know how women can't seem to go to the bathroom unless they are in groups? Since this pole is coming with me to the bathroom multiple times today, I decided to give her a girl's name and think of it like a girlfriend." She started laughing! "Great idea!" she said.

Now every nurse when I get chemo knows already or is quickly told the story of "Jane," who rolls with me to use the restroom. I wanted to find a way to make even chemo not too serious or a downer. In the next chapter, my contributors share stories of how they made each treatment an outing, etc. What can you do to face "Cancer with Joy" even while receiving cancer treatment?

Number Five—Handling the hair loss that comes with "Cancer with Joy."

I am going to share several specific, funny, and real examples of how I handled my hair loss with joy and laughter. Remember there were definitely tears shed. There was certainly sadness. But I did not stay there! I moved from crying to laughing quickly.

To me, hair loss was the most *emotionally* painful moment. The most physically painful moment was definitely when my urologist removed the stent from my right kidney while I was awake and completely aware of what was going on. The doctor's rationale was it would take me longer to come around from anesthesia than the procedure itself, so since it was so quick, why bother with the anesthesia? Well, I certainly wanted to *bother* with it, but my medical team did not see it that way.

Hair loss happened for me in stages. At diagnosis, and as you will see on the website you get access to at the end of this book, I had shoulder-length hair when I was diagnosed and at my first chemo treatment. About four weeks after diagnosis and just a week after my first chemo, we decided to have my hair cut very short. It was probably about as short as it had been in twenty years!

On CaringBridge April 23, 2010, I wrote

I was so pleasantly surprised at how much I like the new very short do! This morning I decided I can't "like" it too much because to fall in love with this & then have it come out... agh! But while we see what the next couple weeks brings this hairstyle will definitely work. My hair is playing the song, "Should I stay or should I go now?" Humor helps along this journey... ☺

I joked that my hair was trying to decide if it should stick around for the rest of the cancer experience or just leave now and come back later!

Number Six—Handling the *hair loss shower* with joy.

I took what I call a *hair loss shower* on May 4, 2010. When I spoke at the American Cancer Society Hope Gala in Lincoln, Nebraska, on March 19, 2011, as a Cancer Survivor Speaker, I had many women come up to me and say, "I too took that shower. I could *totally* relate to what you were saying."

When I wet my hair in the shower that day, I heard a *splat* sound. I had a feeling I knew what it was, and when I looked, *much* of my hair was lying on the tub drain. It had come out when the stream of water from the shower hit my head. I had known this was probably coming because when I would run my fingers through my hair, it would just come out in my hands. It was also coming out on my pillow as I slept at night. I hit the point where I had to vacuum my pillowcase each morning and wash it more regularly because of all the hair on it.

I put shampoo in my hand and went to suds my hair and it just came out in my hands. This is the moment I remember crying the hardest. It is one thing to know something is going to happen, but it is completely different when it actually happens. I have spoken to many women's cancer groups about this because they want a speaker who has had chemo-induced hair loss and has been through what they have or may go through.

Here is how I was able to laugh and find humor even at that most difficult of moments. As a country music songwriter, I listen to country radio most of the time. Here is what I wrote in my CaringBridge for May 6, 2010.

> I was worried about putting my head back under the water & if the rest of my hair would just wash away when my head hit the water stream!! You may laugh, but that thought really enters your mind when all that hair is coming out in your hand. The funny thing is, as I was getting out of the shower with my country radio station on, a song was playing by Reba called "Consider Me Gone." It felt like my hair telling me "Good-BYE!" I started laughing; you just can't make that stuff up! ☺

I remember standing in the shower with shampoo in my hair *agonizing* about the moment I had to put my head back under the stream to rinse. Was the rest of my hair just going to fall out right then and there? Would I be completely bald by the end of this shower? I patted my head after I rinsed and still felt some hair. Not knowing how bad it would look when I looked in the mirror, I put a towel on my head and as I was heading to the mirror to look, I heard Reba singing, "If I'm not the one thing you can't stand to lose… consider me gone!" My hair was the one thing I could not stand to lose; I really REALLY did not want my hair going away, but I knew that was a likely side effect from one of my chemo medicines. This had been covered with me in chemo education provided by my oncologist's office.

Number Seven—The next of many ways I personally handled "Cancer with Joy" was when I completely lost my hair. I handled it with joy by making it fun (for me and others)!

After the hair loss shower in early May, I decided to shave my head so I would not have to take such an emotional shower again. I had visited the local American Cancer Society in April and they loaned me some wigs, hats, and scarves. I also discovered the fabulous "Tender Loving Care" catalogs and ordered some hats, halos, and wigs.

I have handled the complete loss of my hair with joy by having fun with the halos, hats, and wigs. A halo is an elastic ring of hair that gives you the look of having hair with hair hanging down for bangs, on the side, and in the back, but in the heat (as I faced with the Nebraska summer), the coolness of the bulk of your head remaining bald. You cover the bald part with a fun hat! I even involved my friends by doing an online fashion show where I tried on many different looks (various colors, lengths, and styles), had my mom take pictures, and uploaded them to Facebook and my CaringBridge site. I let people "vote" by liking and commenting on their favorite looks to help me choose my best looks for the summer. This let my friends know I was coping with hair loss with joy, actually making it fun and helping them get involved, and having fun with what was happening during my cancer treatment. Of course I will share some of the pictures from this online fashion show with you as part of the bonus that comes with your purchase of this book!

Number Eight—Handling "Cancer with Joy" while dating again.

I was blessed that, in spite of cancer, an old boyfriend came back into my life shortly after I was diagnosed. I met him on my twenty-first birthday—what a present! Thankfully my good friend with me that day was someone who mutually knew both of us, though we had never been introduced. He graduated from the same high school my mom graduated from, and his parents work for the postal service in the area so they have delivered mail to my grandparents and other family members for years! He is the one I mentioned in the first chapter, texting me and seeing me two days before I first heard the word cancer associated with me.

After seeing him *pre-cancer* on March 10, and texting and talking on the phone in March and April, on the phone in May he mentioned it would be fun to come up (he was approximately two hours away) to where I was living so we could do the dinner and a movie thing. I thought that sounded great! I had been involuntarily immersed in this cancer world, and my days were filled with blood draws, pills to swallow, cancer-related fatigue, hair loss, and a feeling of nausea. Not so much fun!

When I told him how wonderful that would be because he was a good friend who I was very comfortable with and had known for years, he clarified, "Well, I'm not exactly asking as a friend." I was so, well, flattered, but also surprised. Did he even know what he was getting into asking a bald cancer patient out on a date? Did he really understand I was BALD at this point? We did not post pictures of me this way on Facebook! That is a personal decision each individual has to make, whether they want to go with their bald head or cover it up. When I looked in the mirror and saw my bald head, I was reminded of what cancer had been able to do to my physical appearance while I was fighting it. I wanted to look "normal, like me."

It was comfortable (cooler in the summer, and less itchy!) to not wear hair around the house, but I wanted to look as much like me as possible when going out. He was used to me with chin- to shoulder-length hair I was sure. That was all gone. Even wearing a wig, would I look like *the me* he had known since 1997 (for almost thirteen years)?

I will talk more about this and about him in the relationships chapter. While we have since broken up for now as we are on different paths in life (him happy in the small town, and me happy in Nashville, which is "not" a small town), he was an important part of my cancer experience in 2010, and is therefore an important part of this book.

The first time we went out again in May 2010, I was wearing a halo and a hat. The halo gave me hair close to my former color, length, and close to a style I had at diagnosis so I felt like "me" and was very comfortable.

Now that you know we started dating again and that he was my boyfriend during those intense rounds of chemo, and even months after I achieved remission, I should tell you more about him. His particular hobby is buying cars on the Internet to fix up and resell. He is as passionate and consumed with it as I am with my songwriting. He has always loved driving fast in vehicles; he is a Pontiac fan specifically. When we met in 1997, we lived about thirty minutes apart and one of the first things he did was bet me how quickly he could get me home. I should have known then what I was getting into!

This is one way I handled hair loss with joy in the midst of rekindling an old relationship. I was at his house one beautiful summer afternoon and we decided to go visit his parents who lived about thirty minutes away. I was wearing one of my wigs that day of course. We jumped in the car, and he proceeded to speed up. He opened the sunroof on the car, and I could feel it happening!

I felt *movement* on my head. He may have forgotten wigs are not stuck to your head like real hair is, but I think he realized it when I clamped my hand to the top of my head, and said, "Hang on hair!" He started laughing!

I could just see my hair getting airlifted *off* my head, sucked up *through* the sunroof, and I would look in the rear-view mirror only to see my hair rolling down the highway! I explained this to him and assured him if that did happen, I would *not* be the one to get out of the car (bald) and chase my wig hair down the highway, but *someone* would! Wigs are not cheap!

We arrived at his parents' house where I had to relay the story that I chose to laugh at, and not get angry over. I never yelled at him for opening the sunroof; it was a beautiful day to let the fresh air in. The funniest part came when his mom offered me a head scarf to tie around my chin to "keep my hair on!" I started laughing at her solution, offering me a head scarf, instead of perhaps telling her son to SLOW DOWN!

Number Nine—Handling "Cancer with Joy" while on an "adventurous" vacation.

The same boyfriend surprised me in July 2010 with an all-expenses paid trip for two that he earned through work to Whistler, Canada. This is where part of the 2010 Winter Olympics had been held. There was another couple he knew going from another store. I knew the other guy and was excited to meet his wife. I had not exactly taken a vacation since being diagnosed with stage four cancer, but luckily the trip fell at a very good time right before the sixth chemo treatment. This is when you are feeling the very best you can at the time because you have had almost three weeks to come around energy-wise.

I had some things in mind I thought would be fun to do on a Canadian vacation, but I knew this was a vacation my boyfriend earned through work, so I waited to see what his ideas for the trip were. I found out I vacation different than my old boyfriend! My idea of vacation is relaxing, but his and the other guy's idea of vacation was, shall I say, adventurous?

On the first full day there, I found myself exploring ziplining! Ziplining is something I personally have *never* had *any* desire to do whatsoever, because I, still as an adult, have a pretty intense fear of heights. Hanging from only a cable whooshing along up high is *not* my idea of a good time. After everything my body and mind had been through in the intense months since diagnosis, I was thinking a massage sounded pretty good! I have never had a couple's massage; I am "saving that" to experience with a very special guy. But it was not my trip and I did not want to spoil the fun for the others. I tried to campaign to do my own thing while they went and did what they wanted to do, and we could all meet up later, but that was unsuccessful!

I am not sure ziplining is for cancer patients who are wearing wigs, but I handled it with joy making jokes out of it as I tried some of the course. When the course got more challenging and higher up, I could handle no more and I "chickened" out of the four-level course. The wife in the other couple joined me in "chickening out" shortly thereafter. We walked the course with the guys up above, shooting pictures and video.

While ziplining, you need to hang on with both hands to steer yourself. I joked that without a hand holding my wig on my head, I was convinced the rush of air would lift my fake hair right off my head! I had a feeling it would fall into the pretty-sounding gurgling stream below, and a bear would waddle up and start eating it! Cracking jokes made me, and those around me, laugh. I hope these specific examples from my personal story inspire, encourage, and show you how you *can* handle cancer, from holidays to hair loss to being in relationships with guys who love to drive fast, with jokes, laughter, and joy. To me, I have saved the best for last with this example.

Number Ten—Co-write a positive song about cancer!

As an aspiring songwriter, I knew a "cancer song" would end up coming out of me, as this experience is now what I know and can write most honestly about. I could not recall hearing a tremendous amount of cancer songs on the radio, even though so many people are impacted by cancer. Everyone knows someone who is a survivor of or is fighting cancer, even if they haven't themselves.

When I went to what my oncologist's office called "chemo education," they handed me a big three-ring notebook called *Your Cancer Care*. One of the tabs in this book is called "Side Effects." This section details all the unpleasant things that the medical team believes is likely to happen knowing what they know about the medicines they are giving you and how they have impacted others. I suppose knowledge is power and they want you to be aware. I remember hearing, "You may have some, none, or all of these throughout the course of your treatment." I joked it would be impossible to have constipation and diarrhea at the same time at least, so not everything could happen at once. Gross, but true!

What I realized as I went through my cancer experience (and you will too) is that, thankfully, not everything that happens is bad. Many, many wonderful, even beautiful things happen. I began thinking how I always find a way to look on the "bright side" of things.

I was working with my tremendously talented co-writer Bob Paterno, and we ended up co-writing the song I am most proud of to date. It merges the "side effects" of cancer treatment with looking on the "bright side." We called it "Bright Side Effects," and yes, you are going to be able to hear it for free as part of the tremendous bonus I have for you at the end of this book.

Here is some of the lyric—

"She said, 'I brought a hat with me to the salon
They took me to the back room with my mom
I couldn't hold back the tears in my eyes
Even my hairdresser cried
But I cracked a joke
With a lump in my throat
That's when I started understanding
What I took for granted
A year ago I didn't bother celebrating 33
Who'd have known that I would be

CHORUS:

Gettin' dizzy blowin' up balloons
For my birthday party we held in a ballroom
Losin' my voice screamin' with joy
Fittin' into that old pair of corduroys
I've got paper cuts from get well cards
And smooth legs
Yeah I found there's bright side effects"

(Huber and Paterno, 2010)

I hope you love this song as much as I have, and that it reminds you, even in cancer treatment, there *are* bright side effects to cancer. There are many positives, if you just look on the bright side and choose to focus on what you have instead of what you do not have! I will share more about this in the emotional fitness chapter. Part of the "Cancer with Joy" brand is offering lots of en'courage'ment. Have you ever noticed before how the word inside encouragement is 'courage?' That is one of many valuable components we offer to you as part of the "Cancer with Joy" (CWJ) community!

In an effort to offer some *additional* value, I said ten ways, but I decided to share *another* bonus way I was able to handle "Cancer with Joy" and it is thanks to a dear friend of mine.

BONUS—Use jokes and humor consistently to lighten the mood and ease tension.

Laughter is so good for you! At community college (in the 90s), I was a member of the drill or dance team that would perform dance routines at half time of football and basketball games. My Drill Team Advisor has stayed a friend all these years, and when she found out about my diagnosis, she began sharing jokes on my CaringBridge guestbook to help me handle "Cancer with Joy" from diagnosis through treatment. Posting these jokes just took a bit of her time and did not cost anything. It was also one of the most appreciated gestures from a friend because it was consistent. She did not just do it once, but just as my cancer treatment went on and on (and still goes on as of this writing), she consistently posted jokes that gave me, as well as others reading my guestbook, a laugh.

I believe these many examples will remind you that there are infinite ways cancer can be handled with joy, humor, and laughter instead of handling it with negativity. I have shared ways I handled "Cancer with Joy." Now I want to share with you some phenomenal stories my beautiful contributors share in the next chapter on how they *also* handled "Cancer with Joy"!

Chapter Three

Ten Stories of "Cancer with Joy"

As the idea of writing a book sharing the "Cancer with Joy" story and much more came to me, I thought it would be terrific to collect stories from *other* cancer patients and survivors to also share with you. I gave you ten specific examples in the last chapter of how I handled "Cancer with Joy." I wanted ten other stories with others' examples of how they too handled "Cancer with Joy" to fill you with ideas and inspiration for how this challenge can be handled! I am thrilled to share stories from men and women, other young adults and those who are older than forty, a mother-to-be going through chemo because she found out she had cancer after she was already pregnant, a story from Ms. Senior America 2009-2010, and even stories of those who gave to *others* volunteering after their diagnosis. EnJOY these additional stories of handling "Cancer with Joy"!

Just Because Cancer Enters Our Lives
Does not Mean Joy has to Exit

By Edward Leigh, MA

"I am sorry to tell you this," my doctor said, "but during the procedure, we found a tumor on your colon." Within a week of hearing those words after a routine colonoscopy, I was in surgery.

From the beginning of this experience, I was determined to maintain my sense of humor and my joy in life. As I contemplated my upcoming surgery, I was concerned that the surgical team's mood may have an impact on my surgery. The last thing I wanted was a bunch of grumpy people opening me up! To guard against this, I felt I needed to give the team a quick motivational pep talk.

Just before the anesthesiologist put me under, I said to everyone, "Please stop what you're doing and turn around. I have a question, 'Does anyone have any issues with anyone else in this room that we need to discuss right now?'" Once I determined that everyone was in a good mood, I turned to the anesthesiologist and said, "You may proceed."

The surgical team knew I would be a handful from the start! I had a clown nose on as I wheeled into the surgical suite. During my weeklong hospitalization, I kept a stash of clown noses in my room. When any members of my healthcare team came to see me, I would not let them do anything to me unless they agreed to one request—wear a clown nose!

The surgery did not remove one part of me—my sense of humor! In fact, the experience heightened my use of humor. I even developed a motto, "Just because cancer comes into our lives does not mean joy has to exit." Armed with this motto, I met the challenges that followed with my fun-loving spirit intact. I even found a new nickname; since I had part of my colon removed, I was now a "semicolon."

My humor helped me cope with chemotherapy side effects. I was having issues with nausea and my healthcare team experimented with a new medication, which my wife delivered to me as I was lying on my bed feeling queasy. On the bottle was written, "Put the pill in the refrigerator for 15 minutes before using." I found those instructions quite strange and since I was feeling so sick, I decided I could not wait to refrigerate. As I was about to swallow the pill, my wife walked into the bedroom and said, "What are you doing? That is a suppository!"

Chemo brain strikes again! (I ultimately did put the pill in the correct place. After doing this, the phone rang. I thought I better answer since it may be my oncologist. It was a lady asking me to sign up for a new credit card. In my chemo brain associated altered state, I told her, "I can't talk now. I have a cold pill in my rear end." She didn't stay on the phone long!)

Throughout my journey, complementary therapies like humor therapy and pet therapy helped me maintain my joy and humor in the face of illness. I set a personal goal for each chemotherapy session: I would walk into each session with a fun prop. Variety is the spice of life so I brought in a diverse array of items such as noisemakers, stress balls, funny teeth, and outrageous hats. I am a bit of a practical joker, so I always made all my chemotherapy sessions a wild time! At one chemotherapy session, I told a nurse that my elbow hurt. She came over to me, and as I was bending my elbow I simultaneously used a hidden noisemaker that made a cracking sound! The look on her face—priceless!

At first, my wonderful oncologist was perplexed by my use of humor. She said very respectfully to me during one visit, "Cancer is so serious, how do you find humor in it?"

I told her, "Cancer is very serious and I am not belittling the serious nature of the disease. However, I am using humor as a coping tool. Some people use music or art as therapy, I use humor therapy."

My oncologist's face lit up and she said, "Now I understand—makes perfect sense."

Actress Annette Funicello once said, "Life does not have to be perfect to be beautiful." Even with cancer, life is beautiful.

Edward Leigh, MA, is the Founder and Director of the Center for Healthcare Communication. He focuses on two areas: helping healthcare professionals effectively communicate with patients, and helping patients take charge of their healthcare. He is a healthcare professional and has worked in the healthcare field for over twenty years. He is a professional speaker, seminar leader, consultant, and coach. He has appeared on The Today Show, The Montel Williams Show, MSNBC News, *the* Discovery Health Channel *and the* Oprah Winfrey Network. *His e-mail is* info@communicatingwithpatients.com *and his website is* www.CommunicatingWithPatients.com.

I Recognized the Choice I Had: Hope vs. Hopelessness

By Gail King, Ms. Senior America 2009-2010

It's been a year since I've been crowned Ms. Senior America, and frankly, I am surprised at how much my life has changed. Previously, I had written about taking back my life after breast cancer and reconstructive surgery. So many women have been asking me what my life is like now, so I thought I would share a few highlights in addition to my promotional appearances on television, radio, magazines, and newspapers.

I am still surprised when I am recognized at airports, train stations, and in restaurants. After marching in the St. Patrick's Day Parade on Fifth Avenue, I was honored meeting with His Excellency, Archbishop

Timothy Dolan, who encouraged my work with support groups. Also exciting was my invitation aboard the USS NY, being honored in Albany by Senator John Flanagan, meeting with former Governor Paterson, and receiving seventeen proclamations this year. Being nominated for Senior of the Year and Suffolk County's Woman's Hall of Fame was a humbling experience. In Washington, DC, I posed on the capitol steps with Bill Livingood, Sergeant at Arms of the House of Representatives, and on Long Island, I also posed with Alec Baldwin at a Carol M. Baldwin Breast Cancer Research Fund Gala, at which I was an invited guest.

What fun I had dancing and speaking at Veterans Centers, chatting onstage with Mickey B, the Prince of Rock and Roll at the Patchogue Theater, crowning State Queens across America, visiting children's hospitals, and making commercials and infomercials. I auditioned and became an extra on *30 Rock*, *Extreme Forensics*, *Royal Pains,* and in the movie *Salt* with Angelina Jolie. *Instant Cast*, a modeling and acting site, follows me around the country in blogs entitled: "Where in the World is Gail King?"

By and far, the most rewarding experiences occur when I speak before support groups including Stony Brook University; Vanderbilt University Medical Center in Nashville, Tennessee; the Pink Ladies Support Group in Mount Juliet, Tennessee; Relay for Life; Strength to Strength program at the Sid Jacobson JCC in Roslyn, New York; Carol M. Baldwin Breast Cancer Research Fund; and Scottish Rites Children's Hospital in Dallas, Texas.

As I stepped outside the box and left my comfort zone, I realized that this has been a year of growth revelations and reflections for me. More than once, I have been asked how and why I would want to share my personal experiences with others. After meeting with survivors aged fifteen to eighty-four, and hearing about their concerns, questions, and lessons in courage, I realized that this was much bigger than I.

I see myself as a symbol of hope and strive to inspire others. If anyone would have predicted that a twenty-five-year-old woman in South Side Hospital who had less than a thirty percent chance of survival would one day be crowned Ms. Senior America, I doubt very few would have believed it. Anything can happen; you must never give up no matter what. The question posed before me should be: how could I not share my story, raise money for cancer awareness, and help the cause? One woman recently said to me: "Your national reign for this year may soon be over, but this is the crown you will wear for the rest of your life."

Included in my motivational presentation is a discussion on early detection and lessons on keeping yourself positive, peppered with personal anecdotes. I share how I refused to become a victim. Instead, I became a survivor, who is actually a victim with attitude, and believe me, I've got plenty of that! I have since become a thriver who has refused to let cancer define me as a person. It's what I had, not who I am.

Early on, I recognized the choice I had: hope vs. hopelessness. I have the power to change my life for the better and to affect the lives of others. Impressed with Winston Churchill's philosophy of never giving up, I included having a positive attitude while combining a balance spiritually, physically, and emotionally. Visualization techniques, prayer, and meditation made me feel relaxed and centered. I also learned the value of exercise in healing. I can still remember squeezing a tennis ball fifty times a day and walking my arm up the hospital wall trying to gain strength on my left side after surgery. I did this for five weeks, and one year later, I won my first doubles tennis tournament at Ocean Bay Park.

Surrounding myself with positive people empowered me in avoiding the negativity and constant tears of those who had given up on me, and those who were subconsciously preventing me from getting well. The seventies had no computers, PDAs (Personal Data Assistants), cell phones, or even cable television. But, I still had a litany of books and medical journals in which I immersed myself as I became my own advocate. By working with my surgeon, I became part of my treatment.

I researched, asked questions, and brought in friends or family during my consultation in case I became nervous or needed to go over what I had been told. This decade had no mammograms, MRIs, or Tumor Markers. Instead, I evaluated and changed my diet, added exercise, sleep, and vitamins.

Just as more rest was needed after surgery, I also needed to get back into my routine. I couldn't wait to get back into my classroom after three weeks in the hospital. My students missed and needed me and that helped. While some cancer patients do not want to discuss their diagnosis or treatment, which must be respected, I actually felt better sharing my journey knowing I was helping others allay their fears. Although I didn't even feel like combing my hair at first, I soon found I felt much better wearing makeup, perfume, and even a gorgeous peignoir as I walked the corridor with my IV machine visiting the children's ward. The children thought I was a princess, as I visited every child I was permitted to see. Giving my flowers away to the elderly patients also filled me with joy as I gave away books (humorous), which friends brought me. Above all else, seeing myself through the eyes of others made me see myself as a symbol of hope and joy in giving back.

Once home, I continued to indulge in bubble baths, humorous books and shows, ate chocolates, had cheerful visitors, pedicures, and milkshakes. You get the idea: spoiling myself really helped.

When William Shakespeare stated, "How sweet are the many uses of adversity," I could only think of all the good that has come from my experience. I was proud of how I handled my situation and I saw my confidence soar as I turned twenty-six years old. I became a more compassionate woman, and realized how much I could learn from the kindness and help I accepted from others. More importantly, I learned how fortunate I was to be able to give back. "Paying it forward" has become an integral part of my life. I learned that you don't have to come in first in a pageant in order to be a winner. A winner is defined in how she lives her life each and every day. I am number one because of who I have become, not because I didn't die. My life is enriched because I am able to help others. I am thrilled to dedicate the second act of my life to volunteering as I am determined to make a difference. I discovered what the humorist Sam Levenson already knew: "You have two hands: one for helping yourself, the other for helping others."

For more information see: www.GailMKing.net.

Be Positive—Like My Blood Type

By Diana Kaaha

Fourteen years ago, my doctor told me I had the worst case of Hodgkin's disease he had seen in fifty years of practice. I had ten tumors the size of grapefruits. The cancer was everywhere—it was time to save my life.

I had a clear choice. I could either see my cancer as an ordeal or an adventure. Lucky for me, I was instantly tossed into the hospital where I found myself fascinated by the whirlwind of activity swirling around me. Adventure easily won!

When I learned my blood type was B+, I knew I had to "Be positive—like my blood type." That became my motto! I refused to listen to negative statistics. I asked my doctor if he had ever seen anyone with my extent of the disease survive, and when he said yes, I told myself, "That's who I will be!"

As scary as chemo felt to me, I couldn't wait to get started. I was sick and misdiagnosed for so long and now chemo was going to end my pain. Nothing could take away the joy I felt knowing that my growing collection of symptoms was finally going to go away. My first chemo day was like a big party just for me.

My body was on a deathbed, but my mind felt energized. I remember the night that put me on the path that saved my life. The nurse assigned to me told me she was one year out from Hodgkin's herself. She was proof that I could survive.

I will never forget her magic words, "Chemo melts Hodgkin's away."

Those words were the catalyst for my first visualization. The melting image became so clear in my mind. It was powerful. My frame of mind changed in a snap.

I felt as if I'd been hired to do a job, and I put the melting image to work right away with the chemo I already had in my body. I imagined hot yellow chemo syrup drenching my cells. I lay in bed with such a huge grin on my face that the nurses asked if I knew the seriousness of chemotherapy.

I was helping myself. I felt I was finally in control. I felt safe—happy!

One image led to another. I began gathering medical information on my disease, until I understood what was happening in my cells and how the chemotherapy would help me get rid of my cancer. I even called upon a cast of characters I created when I was fourteen and created my own unique world of positive visualizations!

I imagined "Chemo Eaters" devouring chemo-covered cells, "Blorts" dancing with my bone marrow to make blood cells, "Slurpants" escorting cancer cells out of my body, "Phuntfish" gobbling up leftover chemo-covered debris, and "Phunts" standing guard over my good cells to protect them from radiation.

I blissfully poured my energy into recreating my own positive healing virtual world on the Web. I shared my progress in a blow-by-blow account of my cancer experience. Illustrating my visualizations became my passion. Thousands of people from around the world responded, cheering for me and telling me I had helped them feel happier and more hopeful about their cancer.

Near the end, during radiation, my platelets plummeted out of control and my treatment was delayed. I felt momentarily mad at my platelets! I knew I had to visualize!

One of my characters, a Slurpant, came to my rescue. I closed my eyes as I watched the Slurpant playfully pull platelets through my bone marrow, creating a current that loosened the platelets off the mother cell. It was easy to do, and I knew it was working. My very next blood test showed an increase in platelets!

Never have I been so proud of my blood. I could not stop smiling!

When it came to my last day of radiation, I wanted to make it joyful and memorable—so I roller skated into treatment. When I rolled into the radiation room, there were balloons from my family streaming up the back of the machine. Everyone in the radiation unit congratulated me as if I was a celebrity—and I felt like one.

To this day, when I look back, I know my positive imagination played a big part in saving my life!

At fifty-five, Diana Kaaha is the author of The Round Diet: Don't be Round, Eat Round, *host of RoundTV (www.youtube.com/roundlady), creator of Roundorama (www.roundorama.com), fourteen-year cancer survivor, former bodybuilding champion (1982-1984), and Silicon Valley information designer who inspires the world to take care of their bodies.* Hello Chemo—A Visualization Survival Guide for Anyone Going Through Chemotherapy *was published in September 2011.*

Giving Joy to Others Helped Me Forget about Cancer

By Elaine Jesmer

My diagnosis was made just a month before Katrina hit the gulf coast, so by the time the rest of the country was mobilizing to help with the recovery, I was deep into treatment. Stuck in the city where I live, I was only able to put in one day as a volunteer for the Red Cross answering questions for Katrina victims. What I wanted to do was "hands on" work, and at the time, that wasn't possible. A year-and-a-half later, when I finished treatment, I asked my oncologist if I was free to roam, and she said "yes." With her okay, and with the financial help of a dear friend, I joined up with a local New Orleans charity and spent two amazing weeks living in a dorm, eating donated food, and working in City Park replanting, cleaning, and riding a bike around the city. Giving joy to others helped me forget about cancer.

I was building something in New Orleans. I didn't see it at the time, but throwing myself into a project that had everything to do with other people, mirrored the beginning of my rebuilding my own life. Thinking solely about others, I surprised myself at what I was able to do, after having spent the past two-and-a-half years juggling operations and dosing my body with some pretty strong drugs and rays. Yet I fit right in with the rest of the volunteers. Nobody had to slow down for me. I could take it, even surviving an attack of fire ants!

Looking back, those two weeks were not only one of the best experiences of my life, but it cleared the decks and allowed me to come home and dive into my life feeling fresh and renewed. I had tossed out the baggage of being a patient, the same way I cleaned the city. Anyone who got on my nerves fell by the wayside. The people who were left were the important ones.

I found it really liberating to completely break away from the environment where I was being treated. Not everybody has the kind of opportunity I had, but "the break" doesn't have to be that dramatic. You can take a bus to the beach for a day (with or without your cell phone), or climb a mountain. I stopped drinking because my cancer had metastasized to my liver, but I didn't miss it. I dumped the car, so now I HAVE to walk; it's not a choice anymore. I got some chickens. Everyone finds what works for them.

Cancer has been a great motivator for me. It's been almost six years since I was diagnosed stage four, and I've never felt healthier. I know some people will think me unrealistic, but I think I lucked out. And I truly believe that if I can make changes in my life, anyone can do it.

You really do get to take back your life.

Elaine Jesmer is the author of "I'm Hot! ... and I'm Bald!": CHEMOTHERAPY FOR WINNERS, available at <u>www.amazon.com</u> and on Kindle. The book and her website, <u>www.elainejesmer.com</u>, offer information and support for getting through the challenge of chemotherapy.

You're the Strongest Person I Know; You Aren't Going Anywhere

By Cristy Norwood, "Warrior Chick"

I remember the night my doctor called me and gave me the news... "I don't know how to tell you this, Cristy, but your biopsy came back showing malignancy. I'm so sorry."

Stunned, shocked, and scared to death (no pun intended!), I remember hanging up the phone and feeling all these emotions raging over me. Breast cancer, me?! I was thirty-six-years-old, newly married, and pregnant with my fifth child—this was not happening to me. My kids needed me, who would make sure they said their prayers at night? Who would love them "to the moon and back"? Who would help them with homework, and cheer them on at their ballgames? I'm the mother, they needed me, the baby I was carrying needed me to bring her into this world, it's my job. I had lost my mother when I was twenty-one-years-old to bone and lung cancer and I still needed her everyday. God would not take me from my babies. Would He?

Six days after the dreaded phone call, I had a PET scan done. I remember lying in the room after they injected me with the dye for my scan, praying to God for His strength and guidance. Asking Him, pleading that the cancer would not have spread anywhere. That He gives me the faith to handle this journey He was about to put me on, with dignity and grace. That He would use me to help others and show them, through me, how cancer can be a blessing. I lay on the scan table and the most calming feeling came over my body, and I just knew it hadn't spread.

My wonderful husband and I went upstairs to the chemo room so I could get fluids to flush out my system, and hopefully keep all the radiation fluid away from my baby girl that I was carrying, and my oncologist called us and said the cancer was no where other than my breast and lymph node area! Praise God! I called my daddy and could hear the relief and tears of happiness in his voice. Two days later I had a double mastectomy and twenty-eight lymph nodes removed (six out of the twenty-eight were malignant), spent four days in the hospital, and came home pregnant and *boobless*. Something about that sounds odd, huh? Ha!

I told myself from day one that I was going to be open and honest with my children throughout this journey. I wanted to share all my emotions, all my procedures, show them my scars, and even let them all (including my then one-year-old) shave my head when that time came. My oldest son Clay and I were talking one day when I had gotten home from the hospital, and he asked me if I was scared (he was twelve-years-old at the time).

"Yes babe, I'm scared. Very scared. Are you?"

To which he replied, "No, I'm not. You are going to be okay, Mom. You're the strongest person I know; you aren't going anywhere."

Wow! Okay, if my twelve-year-old son had that much faith in me and in God, then I needed to as well. So that's what I did, just as I had asked God to do that day I had my PET scan…dignity and grace. Now, to helping others see His graciousness. Thirty chemo treatments, thirty-three radiations, 184 doctor appointments, fifteen surgeries, and birth to a beautiful, healthy baby girl six-and-a-half weeks earlier than her due date, and I feel I've kicked cancer's bootie! I have shared my story step-by-step on Facebook, which has been very therapeutic for me. So "Cancer with Joy"…I feel very blessed to be on this journey still, eighteen months later, and cancer free.

It's an emotional ride and there are days I get down and depressed. There are times I have aches or pains and I think, "Oh my goodness it's back! I have cancer in my toe!" (or whatever is aching at the time). But when I really think about it all, I smile and look at my beautiful family and friends and think how very blessed am I to be surrounded with such love and support. To know that I have been able to touch someone else's life through my experience brings such joy to my heart and lets me know I'm doing just what God has planned for me through this. Changing lives! How could anyone see that as anything other than a reward? There will be many more along the rest of this ride. I look forward to growing old with my wonderful hubby and walking hand-in-hand with him on the beach when we retire. I get to see my daddy play with my children, which I've always thought was beautiful! And I tuck my kids into bed every night, help with homework, go to ballgames, and love them "to the moon and back"! What JOY going through something so life changing can be.

Cristy Norwood lives in the Fayetteville, Arkansas area and is a stage two survivor of Triple Negative Breast Cancer.

Malignant's the Bad One, Right?

By Steve Hilgenfeld, Ordinary Working Dude

So I'm lying around at home feeling like crud, and I decided, "What the heck! Why not go to my doctor so he can send me immediately to the hospital to have my ruptured appendix removed? That sounds like fun!"

Okay, so that's not really how it went, but to reduce the wordiness let's just go with that. So I'm lying there in the hospital two days after being sliced open to have my appendix removed, and the doctor walks in to tell me he got the biopsy back from my appendix and there was a malignant tumor in it. The first thing I said was, "malignant's the bad one, right?"

At twenty-nine, the last thing I thought I would hear is that I had a tumor, let alone in my appendix, which had just been removed. Because it ruptured, it spread the tumor cells all through my abdomen, which they tell me is not a good thing. Luckily there was a doctor only an hour away that specialized in appendix cancer, and he was able to do a right hemicolectomy with HIPEC (heated intraperitoneal chemotherapy) two months after my diagnosis. Basically, they slice you from stem to stern, take out some colon, some lymph nodes, part of your abdominal wall if it has tumors (like mine), and last but certainly not least, your BELLY

BUTTON! All told they took out about 13.5 pounds of flesh. Not the best way to lose weight. At this point, we found out that I was a stage four cancer patient. Let me tell you, the recovery from that surgery was NOT fun, and neither was starting chemo two weeks later. All told I had thirteen rounds of chemo every two weeks, except for a brief period in March when the doctors gave me a break because of a bad reaction to the chemo drugs.

No one ever said chemo was easy, but you're never quite prepared for it. The constant nausea while the drugs work their way through you. The awful taste in the mouth. (I couldn't even drink water, only sport drinks.) The cold sensitivity to the hands, feet, and tongue. Everything I ate was either hot or room temperature. That was pure torture for this ice cream fiend. The weekly blood tests and finger pricks. Oh the finger pricks, how I hated thee!

However, throughout the whole ordeal, one thing remained constant. That was the love of my family, especially my wife who had to put up with my sometimes-crabby butt. She made sure that I wasn't sitting around doing nothing, even though that was (and still is) my favorite thing to do even before I had cancer. She even threw me a surprise thirtieth birthday party and invited all my friends, family, and coworkers. And let me tell you, it was a surprise. With all the support my wife and family gave me, I knew all I had to do was fight this thing and stay strong for them. At twenty-nine, I was determined that this stupid thing called cancer was not going to bring me down. And if it did, I was going to go down swinging. The first thing I said to my doctor (after the stupid question) was "Okay, what do we do now? How soon can I start treatment?" I have cancer. Big whoop. There are a lot of people out there who have it worse than me. I'll take as many drugs as they'll give me, beat this thing, and take on the next challenge in life. Confidence and the willingness to go the distance helped me conquer my fears and anxiety about everything.

My sense of humor helped me the rest of the way. My favorite thing to do right after the big surgery was to lift up my shirt and gross people out. I would tell them that my belly button was gone, but that was okay because I could use it to scare my future kids into behaving. "If you're not good, the belly button fairy will come and take your belly button. Look what happened to me!"

All of this started in September of 2008. I was done with chemo in June of 2009 and have been in remission ever since. I now have a six-month-old son, a wife that still loves my sometimes-cranky butt, and most importantly, the rest of my life to live.

Steve Hilgenfeld is a stage four cancer survivor of pseudomyxoma peritonei originating from appendiceal carcinoma. He currently resides in Lincoln, Nebraska, with his wife and son, and works as a Client Service Manager. Connect with him on Facebook.

How Did I Handle "Cancer with Joy?"

By Hayley Townley

In 2002, I was diagnosed with breast cancer. I was thirty-six. Those three little words, "You have cancer," changed my life forever. I quickly drove to see my doctor to discuss my options. Circling the block to find a place to park, a car directly in front of her office pulled out of its parking space. They even left me time on the meter! I knew it was a sign of things to come.

I was determined to remain the person my friends knew and loved and laughed with/at. I decided to share ALL my experiences with my friends, as well as all who would listen (I'm a blogger). The day my hair fell out as a result of the chemo, I piled my golden locks in the sink, took a photo, then sent it out with the caption, "You think YOU'RE having a bad hair day?!"

Around town, I'm known by my Mustang convertible. The first time I drove down my driveway with the wind blowing through my wig, it ended up in the back seat! My dog thought small furry animals were dropping from the sky and was ecstatic! I had to wrestle it out of her mouth. I found the best way to handle wigs and convertibles was to wear a hat while driving, and a quick wig flip-on when I got to my location. I can't imagine what people thought when I dipped my bald head down out of sight, and then came up with hair.

I had at least eight different colors and styles of wigs, and chose to wear them as an accessory. I was long blonde one day, and short purple the next. Another picture I posted for my friends was me—front and center, completely bald—then a collage of me in my different wigs. The caption was, "I haven't got a thing to wear." I always kept them guessing.

When it came time for my double mastectomy, I chose the DIEP (deep inferior epigastric procedure) flap procedure (they use your stomach fat to make new breasts; if you have not heard about DIEP, you owe it to yourself to check it out). I ate a pint of ice cream every day for a month straight so there would be enough to make me two good size breasts. I lovingly refer to them as Ben & Jerry! I plan on having the best breasts in the nursing home!

I've been given second chances. I looked down the rabbit hole and beat breast cancer. It's joyful how cancer gave me time to figure out what is really important in my life. My husband and I now work together. I spend more time with friends enjoying each other's company, and less time on cleaning my house and working on my "to-do" list. I make time for that vacation—whether that means an afternoon lunch and pedicure with a girlfriend, a romantic getaway with my husband, or a fun-filled trip to Mexico with twenty friends!

I can change a lot of things in my life. Perspective is one of them. You, too, can choose to handle "Cancer with Joy." Go out there and make your own parking space in the universe, and do it with a smile on your face. After all, parking IS an attitude!

Remember: boobs may come and boobs may go, but funny lasts forever!

XOXO, Hayley Townley

Hayley Townley is the creator of www.ThereIsLifeAfterBreastCancer.com, an empowering site for breast cancer survivors and their loved ones, where they can read, write, draw, and share. Its success has prompted a book series, There Is Life After Breast Cancer, *which will be on bookshelves by 2012. Hayley is a spokesmodel for Cleavage Creek Cellars—be sure to check out the 2006 Cabernet Syrah (www.CleavageCreek.com). According to Oprah, Hayley lives in the happiest place in America: San Luis Obispo, California, with her husband, their three dogs, and an extremely lazy cat. She is available for speaking engagements, lives by exceptions—not rules, and can be reached at HayleyTownley@gmail.com. Hayley also throws terrific parties!*

Surprised Joy Amidst a Mother's Struggles

By Jan Hasak

In 1996 cancer splashed into this mother's life. As a busy attorney with three sons, I couldn't fathom at first the dreaded words, "You have breast cancer." After all, my youngest son Josh was only three. But a slow transformation took place as remission replaced clinician.

Mahatma Gandhi once said, "Joy lies in the fight, in the attempt, in the suffering involved, not in the victory itself." I agree. Joy bubbles out more fully when it springs from a well of mourning. In the process of grieving this diagnosis as a young mother, I resolved to replace self-pity with gratefulness. I prepared myself to be "surprised by joy," also the title of a book by C.S. Lewis. And I was determined to find humor at every twist and turn.

My husband Jim brought just that after my lumpectomy when he entered my hospital room, unannounced, with a gift: Rollerblades, with their hopeful eyelets peering up at me. Surprised by joy? You bet! The thought of inline skating when I had surgical drains dangling from my side was ludicrous. It would have bowled me over if I weren't already supine. But a year or so after my chemo daze, I did put them to use (albeit with knee and elbow pads). My two older pre-adolescent boys and I skirted the local park with ease and grace. Well, at least they did.

In a cancer support group for young mothers—a sorority of soul sisters—we connected at a deep level. Among other tidbits, we shared with each other age-appropriate explanations we could use to reassure our children of our continued vigor. Since humor is the only alternative medicine that is not controversial, I sprinkled large doses into our discussion. Even the word for the study of humor, gelotology, brought laughs to these young mothers desperate for an excuse to chuckle. It mustered up an image of geriatrics and Jell-O in this mostly under-forties crowd.

During my second bout with cancer, after each chemo infusion I would sit in my comfy chair at home, nauseated and weak, jotting down my blessings in a journal. Josh, now nine-years-old, peeked in from time to time. After my third round of treatment, he came into my master bathroom bearing a small book.

"Guess what, Mom?" he announced. "I'm writing blessings in my journal, too." And he showed me his little pocket notebook, a birthday favor from a friend. What an extra surprise blessing for me—and all due to chemo!

As a celebratory trip to commemorate the end of chemo treatment, Jim treated me to a trip to Italy. In Turin, we took a leisurely walk to a nearby train station. I had left my breast prostheses at the hotel room. As we looked at the various destination signs we spied a train headed for the town of "Bra." I looked at him quickly and quipped, "Let's not go there." We laughed all the way back to our lodgings, hand-in-hand. Nothing could have brought more merriment to our spirits.

How would I ever have uncovered these treasures without cancer entering my personal space?

Josh is now nineteen and a sophomore in college. After my recurrence, his youth minister had encouraged him to take up the keyboard as an outlet for his emotions. Now he is an accomplished musician in a worship band, a position for which he had to audition. He may never have picked up an instrument if it weren't for his frustration over my cancer plight.

His brothers are college graduates with steady jobs. What a privilege for this mother, faced with a life-threatening illness twice, to live long enough to function as coach, encourager, cook, and field-trip driver to our sons—and then witness two college graduations, with another one soon on the way.

Energized by cancer this mother can actually say she's proud of those "no-hair days." They're a badge of honor. Without them, she never would have breathed in the aromatherapy of unexpected joy that she encountered. And that's an encounter of the preferred kind.

A motivational speaker, patient-advocate, blogger, and author, Jan Hasak shares her story of enduring a breast cancer diagnosis and treatment at age forty-three and again at fifty-two. As an attorney at Genentech, Inc., she wrote patents for over twenty years. She won an award for her account of being treated with its breast-cancer drug, Herceptin®. To find out more about Jan and her inspirational books, Mourning Has Broken: Reflections on Surviving Cancer *and* The Pebble Path: Returning Home from a

Forest of Shadows, visit www.JanHasak.com. You can e-mail Jan at jan@janhasak.com.

Volunteering at a Children's Home Helped Me Face Cancer Treatment with Joy

By Marie Rowe

It never occurred to me that I would one day be diagnosed with cancer. I didn't smoke or drink, was in good shape from regular workouts, and my diet was healthy. Even though there is cancer in my family, no one had suffered from breast cancer. So, imagine my surprise when I was diagnosed with stage two breast cancer at the age of fifty-three.

Since I tend to be a "glass half full" kind of person, my initial response to this news was not one of fear, but an almost matter of fact feeling of knowing I could beat it on my own. Accordingly, I refused the recommended radiation and chemotherapy treatments, and embarked on a series of alternative therapies, which included a macrobiotic diet, Chinese herbs, yoga, meditation, breathing exercises, acupuncture, hypnotherapy…and a positive attitude! My friends and family, although concerned by the route I chose to take, were somehow comforted by my conviction that I could heal myself.

I was extremely disappointed when, exactly a year after my initial diagnosis, I discovered two more malignant lumps in my breast. It was now strongly suggested that I undergo the traditional method of cancer treatment—radiation and chemo—since the cancer was considered aggressive. Rather than reject what I had previously perceived as "poison," I chose to embrace the chemo. I had no idea what it looked like and imagined some kind of torture chamber. Nonetheless, I decided to make an occasion of it and wore make-up, pretty clothes and jewelry, and later lovely hats, whenever I went for treatment. I also read uplifting books and listened to inspirational tapes as I sat in a large comfortable leather chair while the kind oncology nurse gently administered liquid drugs through a vein in my arm.

The first was a clear liquid, which I immediately imagined to be God's light entering my body. Then the red liquid that followed I saw as the color of love. I had no idea I would visualize the treatment in this way, but choosing to, literally, *go with the flow* rather than fighting the disease and resisting the cancer in an aggressive manner, worked for me.

Interestingly, I did not suffer the severe side effects of chemotherapy, as so many women did, and I like to think it had a lot to do with my attitude. I feel that the previous year of alternative therapy also made a difference, and that I had prepared my body to receive the cancer drugs.

When I later had a mastectomy, I was overjoyed to know that I would be getting reconstruction and that my breasts would be reduced in size. I had always envied girls whose breasts were small enough that they could go bra-less, and now I was one of them.

I was not employed during my treatments, but it was important for me to continue volunteering at a children's home several days a week. Whether it was playing in the sand, reading books, or doing crafts, just being in the moment with these abused and abandoned children gave me a lot of joy, and I feel it was a big part of my healing. Simply turning up for these kids made a difference in their lives, and as it turns out, in mine too. I actually received the "Volunteer of the Year" award during this period for my consistency and for organizing drama and craft activities as well as creative writing exercises for the children.

Because I lived alone, a friend suggested I get a kitten for company while I was undergoing treatment. Her cat had just had kittens and a few weeks later, on Thanksgiving, I decided to take home an orange tabby I named Pumpkin. I had no idea that this little furry creature would bring such joy into my life. He was a bundle of love from the very beginning, made me laugh, and was responsible for making me rest. Lying on the couch exhausted from chemo, I would only have to think about getting up to do something, and Pumpkin would race across the room and jump on my chest with his paws around my neck, his face in mine, forcing me to stay where I was. After I lost my hair, I was sitting in bed crying, feeling ugly. Suddenly, Pumpkin jumped up on the bed and draped himself over my head. Not to worry … he would be my hair!

Marie Rowe can be contacted at Mrowe97@gmail.com or 310-479-7219.

Handling "Cancer with Joy"

By Anna Renault

Hearing the diagnosis, "You have cancer!" is never joyous. However, how one handles their disease greatly impacts the journey. Learning to handle the rollercoaster with JOY certainly makes the journey easier.

My journey with cancer began in 1977. At twenty-seven-years-old, I had uterine cancer. Devastated? Yes. I'd been raised thinking cancer meant death; if not death, certainly a long drawn out battle that was horrendously painful. Yet, upon that declaration, I felt relief. This was a diagnosis explaining the craziness—the pain, the bleeding—of what I was experiencing. Then I was told an operation could and would fix things! JOY!

Skin cancer is often considered a minor problem, especially these days; but twenty-five-years ago that dreaded pronunciation "You have cancer!" still sent chills down my spine. Those chills turned to dread when I found out the cancer on my chin were melanoma—a deadly form of skin cancer. My dad lost the tip of his nose to melanoma; I feared losing part of my chin. I didn't! I got a chin lift. The surgeon even kept the scar in the natural crease of my face.

Colon cancer is a silent killer! Getting routine screenings is never pleasant, but with a family history as well as a personal history of cancer, I knew this was something I had to do. And yes, twice cancer cells were found in my colon and were quickly removed.

It is a really wild ride to have received the diagnosis, "You have cancer!" numerous times with different types of cancer. Having just finished twenty-two months of breast cancer, it never ceases to amaze me that life's journey can be so challenging as well as uplifting. So let me answer the question, "How do I handle 'Cancer with Joy'?"

Both as a young woman of twenty-seven and as a fifty-nine-year-old woman, the same thoughts went through my mind, *Lord, you brought me to this. Please carry me through it!* And He has. I've often said the Lord moves in mysterious ways. I am sure a perfect example of that. Throughout the different types of cancer, each bout has strengthened me with purpose to help others facing adversities. I have been blessed to meet new and extremely interesting people. Would I have met some of these fabulous people without cancer? Probably not! Watching and listening to people who have been inspired by my strength to battle these adversities, inspires me to keep doing the best I can with each new challenge. Seeing people's attitude change, their knowledge growing, and their awareness being raised has given me joy in my heart to know that my life has had such an impact on so many.

Family and friends have often said, "Anna you are strong!" Co-workers and fellow parishioners comment that my story is inspirational to them. I often hear people say they have stopped moaning and groaning about minor aches and pains or little bumps-in-the-road-of-life after hearing my medical history. Medical personnel are often in awe of the extent of my medical issues, which seems to spur them on to provide super-great care for whatever the current problem of the day might be. Recognizing these things gives me joy!

So, as a young woman of twenty-seven with cancer, I made a conscious decision to live my life to the fullest. Not knowing when my last day on earth might be, I chose not to let cancer rob me of a full and exciting life. Yes, I have had days when my body aches so badly that it's painful to simply relax in a bath with Epsom salts! Yes, I've had days when I've cried myself to sleep too many times to count in a twenty-four-hour period. And yes, I've had numerous and unusual side effects from chemo and radiation therapy. However, there have also been the upsides throughout the struggles. I actually compiled many of them in chapter 16 of my book, *Anna's Journey: How many lives does one person get?* (*e.g.,* Teaching the doctors a few things! Getting people to pray!)

Learning to celebrate all the little things will give you joy! Learning to appreciate a bird eating crumbs on your windowsill, spending extra time with family and friends, closely watching the blossoming of a flower, or identifying all the shapes one sees in the clouds will fill one's heart with gladness.

Knowing that I have yet another day to live, love, and make a difference, gives me joy!

Anna Renault lives on the east side of Baltimore County, Maryland, and is a survivor of multiple cancers and tumors: uterine, colon, ovarian, skin (melanoma & squamus), and breast.

Bonus Years

By Lois Hjelmstad

In 1990, the night before my first mastectomy, I wept as I poured out a poem, "Goodbye, Beloved Breast." As I dealt with the many issues facing me, poems continued to spill onto paper. I showed about twenty of them to my oncologist and he said, "You must do something with these." Easy for him to say.

Nothing was easy for me. A year earlier, on a bright April morning when I was feeling especially well and happy, I had felt as if I could conquer the world. That afternoon chills shook my body and by bedtime I had a temperature of over 104 degrees. The high fever eventually resolved but I continued to run small fevers, ache from head to toe, and fight extreme exhaustion. Five months later I was diagnosed with chronic fatigue syndrome (CFS). At age fifty-eight I had become interminably ill and now at fifty-nine I had breast cancer.

My surgery and the five weeks of daily radiation therapy tired me even further. My husband, Les, and I had planned a trip to Europe that summer, but treatment had to come first. I suspect I would have liked Europe better.

To quell our disappointment a bit, Les suggested that we make each afternoon trip to the radiation center into a little outing—one day we stopped for an ice cream cone, another day we sat on a bench in the park and soaked up the sunshine, on another we stopped briefly at a department store and he insisted I find a pair of earrings. Every day he thought of something that I would have enough strength to do.

Fourteen months later, the doctors amputated my remaining breast. I felt a great sense of urgency at that time, so Les and I made sure our affairs were in order. Then, remembering the admonition of my oncologist, I pulled out all of the poems I had written about cancer, as well as those I had written earlier. I spent that summer, fall, and winter adding entries from my diaries, reflections, and photos. By the summer of 1993, I had a book: *Fine Black Lines: Reflections on Facing Cancer, Fear, and Loneliness.* And I had found comfort, healing, and joy in that project.

But I found even more joy in what happened next. I began speaking to groups of survivors, healthcare professionals, and others. People told me over and over that my words were helping them, and bringing them hope. Since then my husband has driven over 400,000 miles as I have spoken more than 575 times in all fifty United States, Canada, and England. (We flew to England, of course.)

On my next birthday I will be eighty-two. I have been granted a longer life than I had any reason or right to expect. I had the opportunity to be with my mother as she struggled with non-smoker lung cancer. I had the years I needed to finish the book I began writing for her soon after she died on Mother's Day five years after my own cancer diagnosis. Once again, writing moved me beyond regret and despair into acceptance and peace. On our fiftieth wedding anniversary, I promised Les that I would write our love story for him. I have had time to complete that book.

Cancer is ugly. I certainly wish to acknowledge my numerous friends who have valiantly fought the disease and lost the battle. I will always remember their lives, honor their struggle, and draw strength from their courage.

But for those of us who are given bonus years—however many—cancer brings a gift of deepening awareness and immense gratitude. I greet each new dawn as if it were the First Morning.

Lois Tschetter Hjelmstad is the author of Fine Black Lines: Reflections on Facing Cancer, Fear and Loneliness; The Last Violet: Mourning My Mother, Moving Beyond Regret; *and* This Path We Share: Reflecting on 60 Years of Marriage. *Her website is* www.facingbreastcancer.com *and she can be contacted at* hjelmstd@csd.net *or 303.781.8974.*

I am not sure if you were counting, but I said this chapter was ten stories of how others handled their cancer experiences with joy, and then I snuck an extra one in as *another* bonus for additional value. In my next chapter, I want to give you a dozen recommended dos and don'ts at diagnosis from my personal experience of having been there. I did not "do" some of the dos. I definitely did some of the don'ts though because no one told me not to, and I hope you can benefit from my experience through your reading of "Cancer with Joy."

Chapter Four

Twelve (Recommended) Dos & Don'ts at Diagnosis

There are definitely more dos and don'ts you will hear about at diagnosis, but I know from personal experience, that moment and the time immediately following can feel extremely overwhelming! I want to share a dozen dos and don'ts I personally feel are very important to consider right away. Several of them take virtually no time at all.

Number One—DO get a second opinion/ go to someone who makes you comfortable!

I think it is very natural to feel shock and disbelief at diagnosis. I certainly was not expecting to hear I had cancer at the young age of thirty-three! A second opinion will definitely help give you peace of mind that there is no mistake, and that two medical doctors have reached the same conclusion.

Earlier, I briefly mentioned my story of the ENT (Ear, Nose, and Throat) specialist my general physician sent me to who I could not stand!

I am easy-going and friendly and get along with virtually everyone, so it was surprising to me to have this strong of a reaction. *Dr. Arrogant* had absolutely no bedside manner working with patients and families. My mom was with me at this appointment, and she asked a question he must have thought he already answered. Well, excuse us if we did not hear your every word because our heads were spinning just a little!

Dr. Arrogant looked down at her through his glasses way down at the tip of his nose and said something like, "Well-l-l-l, my SECOND answer will be the same as my FIRST!" and acted as if he was wasting his breath repeating himself. No patience, no compassion, no more visits to Dr. Arrogant! I began asking around and a friend of mine knew of another ENT. That was the doctor who would make a slit in the right side of my neck and remove a lymph node mass on April Fools' Day! It is your diagnosis, and your body. Go to whom you want!

I hit it off immediately with my oncologist to whom I was sent to see on March 26, 2010 less than forty-eight hours after my diagnosis was confirmed. If I would not have, I *definitely* would have looked around for someone else. When you think about the amount of time you will spend with your doctors and how personal you have to be with them, you have to feel comfortable with them!

My oncologist made me even more comfortable with him by suggesting I go to see another doctor at UNMC (University of Nebraska Medical Center) in Omaha, Nebraska, to confirm the treatment plan he was prescribing (six rounds of five different chemotherapy medicines, each spaced three weeks apart). I went to UNMC in May and again in September to see this second lymphoma specialist. All results from tests I had done (CT scans, PET scan, bone marrow aspirations, etc.) would be copied to multiple doctors. I was asked where I wanted the results sent when I registered or checked in, and I just went down the list because with stage four cancer, I had quite a few doctors on my team!

If your oncologist does not volunteer this, I would recommend you ask, "Who else could I go see to confirm this diagnosis and to give their opinion on our proposed treatment plan?" This is also where you could use the phone book (if anyone uses those anymore!), or Google for oncologists in your area to get a listing. Check out their websites and/or call them directly. Ask others you know for referrals.

Number Two—DO get mad, sad, bitter, depressed, etc.

Feel the emotions you are naturally feeling. Don't try to suppress or fight them off. I believe you need to experience what you are feeling. I have sobbed being grateful for *big* boxes of Kleenex to wipe my eyes and blow my nose. Let it out! I have said several times at "Cancer with Joy," we realize no one is happy they have cancer. I was hardly pleased to get my diagnosis!

I know that while reading this you may be thinking, "WHAT? Isn't this book about helping me handle 'Cancer with Joy'?" Yes, it is, and that is why I propose you consider setting a timeframe and as you start accepting your diagnosis that you don't *stay* mad, sad, bitter, and/or depressed. Realize that you have tremendous power as you can *choose* to look for the "bright side effects" I mentioned earlier.

When the hair on my head fell out in the hair loss shower, guess what? It also didn't grow back on my legs or under my arms. I shaved and then had perpetually smooth, soft, even silky, and very sexy legs and that was definitely a "bright side effect!"

I chose to laugh at the fact that it was now easier than it had ever been for me to change my look. On a chilly day, I could pull on my shoulder-length hair wig, but on a hot day where I would have had my normal hair up off my neck I could wear a short wig or just a hat!

I chose to make the hair loss fun instead of only crying over it. *That* is moving beyond sadness to having "Cancer with Joy!" That is what I want for you. I am here to help you throughout your journey. This book doesn't say "The End" at the end. That is because it is only the beginning of me being there for you through this.

I have experienced stage four cancer; I went through chemotherapy and had hair loss. I discovered how to handle it all with joy and since no one in the world has ever come forward to teach this idea of "Cancer with Joy," (I was personally shocked the domain was available) I am here for you to help you handle it with joy too!

Number Three—DON'T panic.

Okay, I know personally, this is easier said than done. Try not to panic. Be comforted with this fact: cancer is certainly not always the quick death sentence it used to be. I am speaking from being diagnosed with stage four cancer too. I have said before, there is not a stage five. I remember when I found out my diagnosis and we were learning exactly what stage it was, meaning where all the cancer was, and exactly what type of lymphoma I had (Hodgkins, Non-Hodgkins, more specifically what sub-type, I had Follicular), I tried to reassure myself by the fact that I felt fine and surely it couldn't be further than stage one or stage two at the highest.

When we found out it was in the bone marrow, and the kidneys (major organ involvement), I felt some panic. I reminded myself, though, of all that can be done these days. The panic tidal wave washing over me subsided. My paternal grandfather was diagnosed with lung cancer around Christmas in 1986 and he passed by the next June.

Of course, we are all going to die one day. Not a pleasant thought, but if you live, you will someday pass on. A cancer diagnosis merely forces us to face our eventual mortality often unexpectedly. It is not comfortable. But I was comforted greatly as I educated myself about all that *can* be done with a cancer diagnosis and for treatment these days.

Number Four—DON'T go to the Internet as your primary, initial source of information.

I can recommend this after doing this. I am hoping to save you the anguish and pain I put myself through unnecessarily. Google is my friend—I thought! As a member of "Generation X" (born in 1976), I Google everything and am totally infatuated with how quickly more results than one person could possibly go through are returned to me. Knowledge is power I have always heard; so much knowledge available upon a click must equal tremendous power!

On Friday, March 12, 2010, when my general physician mentioned the word "lymphoma" to me as a worst-case scenario, where did I go that Friday night? I was single at this point, but it was not out on a date. I was googling! I was freaking myself out is what I was doing. I did searches like, "How quickly does lymphoma KILL?" Something showed up that said, "Yes it could if left undiagnosed and without treatment." Now, did I focus on it COULD or the without treatment part? No! I focused on yes! Yes it could kill!

I also found this on the Internet! Can Hodgkin's lymphoma kill? "Answer: yes it does, I know a lot of people that have dies from it and very few survive." The typo (dies instead of died) would probably clue you in there as to how credible this information is, but reading this will put fear into people unnecessarily!

Here is the problem with both of the above. *Who* provided this information? What are their credentials? Where did they go to medical school? When you begin googling questions, clicking on results, and reading whatever you find without finding out or considering the source, you are really opening yourself up to the possibility of receiving a lot of inaccurate information that could terrify you unnecessarily.

Anyone can be a content provider these days. Anyone with a computer and Internet access can go to any of the many free blogging websites, create a blog, and begin distributing content in minutes upon deciding they have something to say about anything. Depending on how adept they are at adding tags and search engine optimization, their content could show up rather high in search results. We should know by now just because we read it in print that does not mean it is true, but too many times we believe, and we believe the worst.

I had almost two weeks, or twelve pretty agonizing days between when I first heard the words "lymphoma" and "cancer" associated with me on March 12, and when I confirmed my cancer diagnosis on March 24. The only doctors I saw during this time were my general physician and Dr. Arrogant, who I did not see again. I had a CT scan on March 12, and an ultrasound needle biopsy on March 19. I did not see my oncologist for the first time until March 26. That is a long time to be googling and terrifying yourself when you don't need to be. How about doing especially the next two *dos* instead?

Number Five—DO designate your primary caregiver(s)/team.

Who will attend most if not all of your appointments with you and be by your side? Stay away from googling questions and think about and decide this!

As an unmarried woman at diagnosis, my choice was my mom. Your primary caregiver could be your spouse, roommate, sibling, adult child, parent, close friend, neighbor, or someone else not even mentioned. You could have a team of people versus just one person who take turns helping with needs and taking you to appointments. This is definitely something to decide as early on as possible. Make sure that person or those people know their role. "I'm planning on you to be my primary caregiver throughout this and want to make sure you accept the responsibilities that will go with that role. <Detail said responsibilities: coming with me to appointments, grocery shopping, meal preparation, drying my tears!> Can I count on you?"

Number Six—DO write all those questions down!

If I've told you to stay off the Internet and to designate your primary caregiver(s), then you may wonder what you *are* supposed to do with the many, many questions swirling around in your head. You will ask these of the doctors you see during initial consultations, etc.

Don't try to rely on your memory to hold all these important questions, as your mind is so overwhelmed. Do log all your questions in a notebook. I was relieved to go to appointments with a comprehensive list of questions I had thought about. I fired them off at my medical professionals, as they needed to keep moving with their full patient load but would always say, "What questions do you have?" I could just roll down my list, make notes of their responses, and not worry that I had forgotten something. It is a terrible feeling to have your medical professional in front of you and not be able to remember your question. Inevitably, it will come to you, after they have gone on to their next patient! Be prepared with a list of your questions. I would even ask the exact same question of both doctors. I got opinions from both to listen for consistency or variances in their responses.

This is where it is also very helpful to have your selected caregiver or someone with you at appointments. Often I would visit with the doctor while my caregiver scribbled notes. There were appointments where both of my parents attended, and we even brought our camcorder and asked permission to record the appointment so I could watch it again later! This was very helpful as then I had my doctor's words, but could also see their body language and hear their tone as to how they answered my question. As I have taught for years as a professional trainer, the real meaning of communication is in so much more than just word choices!

Another idea would be to bring a pocket digital recorder with you and ask their permission to record the appointment so at least you could hear exactly what they said and how they said it later on.

Number Seven—DO decide how you will keep "the masses" informed.

I confirmed my diagnosis on Wednesday, March 24, 2010, and by Saturday morning, March 27, 2010, I had started my free *CaringBridge* website. My mom knew of someone who had used CaringBridge and was able to pass this free valuable resource along to me. It is my hope that you have bought or been given this book as soon after your diagnosis as possible and you may have fast-forwarded to this chapter to see the recommended diagnosis dos and don'ts. I hope you will establish a CaringBridge or other site like it (see the resources chapter for more ideas) quickly after your diagnosis too. It will save you an incredible amount of valuable time and definitely precious energy throughout your cancer experience.

As I updated Facebook and sent mass text messages to friends to let them know "what was going on," all the comments and questions on Facebook and voice mail messages on my cell suddenly felt very overwhelming to deal with. I was very touched to know so many people cared and understood their curiosity and questions, but it took so long to share the exact same information one person at a time. I made phone calls and annoyed myself repeating the same thing I had just told someone except I was now speaking to someone different.

There has to be a better way I thought! Facebook is one great tool but, just like Twitter, status updates (and tweets) are limited in characters! My CaringBridge site is now over a year old. I was able to create my story bringing everyone up-to-speed rapidly on how we arrived at a confirmed cancer diagnosis, add journal entries, and even share photos. (Remember the online fashion show when I shaved my head! I put pictures on

Facebook and CaringBridge and solicited others' input to get them involved!). Plus there is a guestbook people can sign to leave messages of encouragement for you.

Another thing I love about CaringBridge is that you can set levels of security on your site. After all, you are blogging about personal things and sharing your private health information. You have the option of low to high privacy settings. I had all visitors to my site log in. This allows me to create some amazing reports of who has visited my site. Some people *never* signed my guestbook, but, thanks to the privacy settings I could control, I know they were there reading!

Since I set-up my site within seventy-two hours of my diagnosis, I immediately began saying on Facebook that the CaringBridge site was the place to go to get information. My friends definitely understood I couldn't take the time and energy to call them and repeat the exact same thing over and over, one at a time. They learned CaringBridge was the best place to go to get the latest! Even if you can't update it, you can designate someone (that primary caregiver, etc.) who can do it for you!

Number Eight—DON'T try to handle everything alone.

While this is somewhat obvious, I have talked with too many cancer patients who have said they do not want to be a burden to anyone. As an independent woman, I definitely understand the desire to "do it all yourself," but this is a time when others certainly want to help you and feel as if they have been able to do something for you. Let them! I would also recommend here that you keep a paper or computer list of tasks and things you need, so that you don't forget things.

I received so many cards in the mail, voice mails, and calls, and people I spoke with that said, "What do you need?" "If you think of anything you need, just let me know." "Don't hesitate to call." "Let us know what we can do for you." Don't be afraid to tell them when they ask! People who care for you want to feel useful. In the resources chapter I will tell you about an amazing resource called Lotsa Helping Hands that organizes help in times of need.

Number Nine—DO talk to someone who has "been there."

This is so helpful! Part of my passion in writing and getting this book to you is that you are able to learn from my experience and won't make mistakes I made, because you have me, who is further down the path since diagnosis. I will share more about this specific resource that I found out about later than I would have liked to, but I would recommend you sign up with *Imerman Angels* immediately. Their website, www. imermanangels.org, says, "Imerman Angels carefully matches and individually pairs a person touched by cancer (a cancer fighter or survivor) with someone who has fought and survived the same type of cancer (a Mentor Angel)." I now am signed up to volunteer with them so you could receive a personal phone call from me!

There are thankfully several groups out there providing one-on-one cancer support. My goal is to save you time and energy by telling you about these groups in the resources section of this book versus you having to search for them on your own when you have other more important things to be doing! It is my purpose to help you handle this with joy by making it easier for you!

Along with talking to someone who has been there, I would definitely recommend you call the American Cancer Society and your related cancer group. What I mean by this is I had lymphoma so I contacted the LLS (Leukemia & Lymphoma Society). If you have breast cancer, you could contact komen.org and click on "I've been diagnosed with breast cancer" in the upper left corner. You could also click, "Someone I know was diagnosed." If you have been diagnosed with cervical cancer, you could go to www.nccc-online.org, the National Cervical Cancer

Coalition. Their first goal listed is to "maintain an on-going support system for women, family members, and friends facing issues related to cervical cancer, HPV, and other HPV cancers."

Number Ten—DO control what you can.

This idea gave me great comfort because I knew some things would be out of my control. I decided right away to try not to worry about things that were out of my control. After all, I could make myself physically sick worrying about things that I could do nothing about. Why bother doing that? When I began worrying about things, I would immediately ask myself, "Is it within my control?" If the answer was yes, I thought what I could do about it instead of what I could not do. If the answer was no, I tried to focus my time and precious energy on things I could control.

Let me give you an example. Because I had shoulder-length hair, hair loss was one of the first things I heard and wondered about, especially as a woman. I am not suggesting at all that hair loss is easy if you are a man, but I have told you before, my hair loss was the most emotionally painful moment for me. I decided at diagnosis I would maintain control over what I could, and I was always pretty sure if my hair started coming out, I would control that by shaving my head. I would control how it came out and exactly when I went bald.

Now that I think about it, *that* may have been why I cried so hard during the hair loss shower. It was because I was not in control; it felt like it was happening to me! Deciding I would shave my head gave me a sense of peace in that it would happen on my terms. Making the choice to look on the bright side, I focused on what I would save on not needing haircuts approximately every six weeks, shampoo and conditioner, and styling products. Not to mention all the time it took to wash my hair (I have always enjoyed long showers!), blow dry it, and style it.

I became so used to simply throwing on a wig or whatever look I wanted for the day now that my hair has begun growing back, I often still throw a hat on over my very short hair and go. I have many pictures online of me in a hat still because I grew so appreciative of the time saved on styling hair with a curling iron, etc. I do not have that time built back into my schedule yet. It was actually nice!

Number Eleven—DO try to keep a sense of normalcy to life.

I mentioned the first full week after I was diagnosed I had a daily appointment for an initial consultation, physical, or surgical procedure! My calendar rapidly filled with appointments, consultations with specialists, tests, follow-up on test results, chemo treatments, Neulasta® (white cell booster) shots automatically the day after every chemo treatment, etc., etc. I am all for anything you can do or keep in your life to still feel normal. As creatures of habit, we are generally somewhat resistant to change, and if we can keep some routine things routine, it provides a sense of calm.

Ask your medical team for sure, but could you keep your workout schedule? Yes, probably, with some modifications. Just listen to your body if you feel fatigued or nauseated. Can you still go to cooking class? Could you keep your monthly pedicure appointment? Can you meet the guys for a beer on Friday night?

If everything in your life changes, that will be difficult to adjust to, especially coupled with physical changes you see as you move along in your treatment plan and all the different emotions you feel. Try to keep some things that were on your schedule before cancer, as things on your schedule after diagnosis.

Number Twelve—DO plan to attend a *Look Good...Feel Better* class.

Look Good...Feel Better is a national collaboration of the Personal Care Products Council Foundation, American Cancer Society, and the Professional Beauty Association/National Cosmetology Association.

At www.lookgoodfeelbetter.org it says, "Helping Women with Cancer," so the men reading may be wondering what is for them. But I found *Look Good...Feel Better for Men* for you too! At lookgoodfeelbetter. org/programs/programs-for-men it says, "Look Good...Feel Better for Men is a practical guide to help men deal with some of the side effects of cancer treatment—skin changes, hair loss, stress, and other issues." This resource is also available to teens. I will talk more about it in the resources section.

I was diagnosed at the end of March and attended my *Look Good... Feel Better* class in June. While I can't say I went immediately, I attended the first month after I shaved my head. I was getting comfortable with hair loss and accepting the possibility of eyebrow loss (we were taught how to draw eyebrows!). I still believe this is a "do" right at diagnosis because I believe having this scheduled on your calendar, even if you don't attend right away, will truly give you something to look forward to. The classes are free, you will meet some terrific people who both teach these classes and attend them, and you will come away with a fantastic goody bag full of free products! It was a wonderful experience overall.

Number Thirteen (BONUS)—DO consider fertility if you are in the age range you could conceive children and you think you may want them one day.

This is one "do" I did not do, and I hope to help you through my experience. We moved so quickly—it was three weeks to the day from when I confirmed my cancer diagnosis to when I was receiving my first chemo treatment, but no one talked to me about preserving fertility. I do not feel like child-bearing is out of the question for me now, no one has told me it is not, but if I do meet Mr. Right and become interested in having children, I will need to consider what chemo medicines have been administered to me and subsequently my eggs. It may have been easier to have preserved eggs before chemo. I share fertility information in the resources chapter.

I hope you find this list, compiled from my personal experience, very helpful in giving you things to do and to try not to do immediately at diagnosis. There are plenty of other dos and don'ts in time, but so as not to overwhelm you during a time when you are already feeling some of that, a dozen tips will get you started very nicely. It will help you to feel a sense of calm by having a manageable list of initial dos and don'ts.

Chapter Five

Your Cancer Diagnosis & Healthcare Reform

This is the toughest chapter for me to think about and write. I believe that is because it is the most controversial chapter. Often controversy arises from simple misunderstandings, and when there is clear, respectful communication, controversy can be cleared up. This chapter is so important for me to write to add my real personal experience as a stage four cancer patient and the founder of "Cancer with Joy" to the dialogue.

Ironically, President Barack Obama signed the Patient Protection and Affordable Care Act, better known as healthcare reform, into law Tuesday, March 23, 2010. I received confirmation of my cancer diagnosis the *very* next day! At the time of my diagnosis, I was uninsured. I want to share with you what the healthcare reform bill signed into law in March of 2010 means if you are: also uninsured at the moment of your diagnosis, or if you are currently insured.

At www.empowher.com, an article titled, "What Healthcare Reform Means to Cancer Survivors" by Pat Elliott begins, "Cancer survivors in the United States have typically faced two key stressors at the same time: dealing with their illness while also trying to survive the crushing financial burdens that come with it, regardless of their personal insurance status." I agree with "crushing financial burdens." Crushing is definitely not too strong of a word.

Unfortunately, every place I went, and the number of places literally exploded as I saw (this list is *only* from the first few weeks): my general physician, a hospital for the CT scan, Dr. Arrogant the first ENT, another hospital for the ultrasound needle biopsy, my oncologist, back to an aforementioned hospital for a PET scan, a second ENT, a urologist, back to my general physician for a physical to get cleared for surgeries, to a new hospital to have the surgery that removed "Dick" the lymph node to test the mass, and back to the hospital where "Dick" was removed to have the stent placed from the bladder into the right kidney. I have not even gotten into follow-up appointments, getting a bone marrow aspiration done to test the marrow, having the port placed, and then getting into the chemotherapy treatments themselves, blood draws, *and* Neulasta® shots!

You get the point, which is there were a *lot* of places I was suddenly going and every single place wanted my insurance card, of course, right away, up-front, before any care was given. I had to tell them I was uninsured. In addition to the incredible stress of a stage four cancer diagnosis, I feared going to the mailbox where bills dominated over the get well and thinking of you cards that were coming. Places I hadn't even been to and people I had never seen in person billed me for testing a mass, etc. I speak confidently when I say the amounts on these bills would overwhelm and stress out virtually all of us except the very, very richest of the rich. I kept thinking, *No one asks to get sick, of course, and no one is guaranteed they won't get cancer as it does not discriminate and can strike anyone at anytime.*

Now that I was diagnosed with cancer I figured my likelihood of getting insurance (pre-reform taking effect) was low, but I needed to at least try. Sure enough, I applied in April 2010 and was denied. As an expense versus a profit center paying monthly premiums that couldn't touch what I needed to have paid out, no insurance company that is in business *to make a profit* was going to insure me.

That is until healthcare reform passed! What you need to know if you are uninsured like I was at diagnosis, is at www.whitehouse.gov/ healthreform/relief-for-americans-and-businesses#healthcare-menu where it states, "Uninsured Americans with preexisting conditions can get insurance through the new Pre-Existing Condition Insurance Program (PCIP)." This is at www.pcip.gov and I will talk about this further in the resources chapter as well. At www.pcip.gov it states, "The Pre-Existing Condition Insurance Plan makes health insurance available to people who have had a problem getting insurance due to a pre-existing condition." Later it states, "You must have a pre-existing condition or have been denied coverage because of your health condition." Yes, someone was finally speaking about health insurance to me, the undesirable cancer patient!

According to www.healthcare.gov/law/timeline/index.html#event1-pane, this is a "national program established July 1, 2010… This program serves as a bridge to 2014, when all discrimination against pre-existing conditions will be prohibited."

I will save you time searching and share in the resources chapter additional valuable sites I wish I had known about sooner that could offer financial assistance. I do not want to turn this chapter into a list of websites, but rather share some facts about the healthcare reform from mainly government websites to help you understand the many good things it will mean for you as someone newly diagnosed with cancer or knowing someone diagnosed.

For parents of children newly diagnosed, you need to know that at www.whitehouse.gov/healthreform/healthcare-overview#healthcare-menu it says, "The new law prohibits discriminating against children with pre-existing conditions. Before reform, tens of thousands of families have been denied insurance each year for their children because of an illness or pre-existing condition. New rules will prevent insurance companies from denying coverage to children under the age of 19 due to a pre-existing condition."

The www.empowher.com article I referenced earlier by Pat Elliott also says, "The National Coalition for Cancer Survivorship (NCCS), a leading non-profit cancer advocacy organization, has praised the passage of the healthcare reform bill. NCCS says the bill includes key provisions that protect patients, bringing America's 12 million cancer survivors and the 1.5 million more that are diagnosed each year closer than ever to getting the quality of care they need and deserve."

What about if you have insurance when you receive your diagnosis? The majority of Americans do have health insurance. I want to share some statements from government websites about what healthcare reform means for you. This is good news!

At www.whitehouse.gov/healthreform/healthcare-overview#healthcare-menu it says, "The new law bans dropping your coverage when you need it most. Before reform, insurance companies could cancel your coverage when you were sick and needed it most because of a simple mistake on your application. Under reform, this practice will be prohibited."

"The new law restricts the use of annual limits. Insurance companies' ability to place annual limits on care will be restricted." In addition to annual limits, I found where "the new law bans lifetime limits. Before reform, cancer patients and individuals suffering from other serious and chronic diseases were often forced to limit or go without treatment because of an insurer's lifetime limit on their coverage. Insurance companies can no longer put a lifetime limit on the amount of coverage enrollees receive, so families can live with the security of knowing that their coverage will be there when they need it most."

The healthcare.gov/law/timeline site I referenced earlier in this chapter also states, "eliminating lifetime limits on insurance coverage is effective for health plan years beginning on or after September 23, 2010. Under the new law, insurance companies will be prohibited from imposing lifetime dollar limits on essential benefits, like hospital stays."

This chapter is very brief because healthcare reform is a very new law, and, with so much misinformation out there confusing individuals, it is unfortunately misunderstood to be a bad thing. I fully expect additional debate of this bill that has been signed into law, reform of our broken in places healthcare system, and additional laws affecting health insurance companies to be passed. With that thought, I did not want to create a substantial chapter in the book on this topic that would become outdated as the bill that has been passed is added to.

I will certainly come back to the topic of your cancer diagnosis and share additional financial resources that could be of assistance in the resources chapter. I believe any comprehensive cancer book for the newly diagnosed should have a financial piece to it. Finances are a significant piece of the puzzle for the newly diagnosed, just as emotions are. (Both finances and emotions are addressed in several places throughout the book.)

In the resources chapter, I will share about websites like www. giveforward.com. "GiveForward pages empower friends and family to send love and financial support to patients as they navigate a medical crisis. Create a page today to spread hope and contribute to a loved one's out-of-pocket medical expenses," it says on their home page. This chapter was intended to focus on simply what healthcare reform will mean for the newly diagnosed with cancer, whether they are uninsured (as I was) or whether they have health insurance.

Chapter Six

Cancer & Your Relationships

Considering there are whole books out there on relationships, I certainly want to devote an entire chapter here to relationships as they relate to a cancer diagnosis. In this chapter, I discuss both personal and professional relationships.

Professional relationships on your job or in your business (such as in my case as a self-employed professional speaker and individual coach) include: talking to your boss, co-workers, employees, customers, suppliers, and others you know professionally through associations, etc. I also think a discussion on professional relationships should include your new team of medical professionals. Personal relationships include: spouse or partner, boyfriend/girlfriend, whoever's in your family circle (parents, grandparents, children, grandchildren, siblings, aunts, uncles, cousins), and friends.

When thinking of your new professional relationships with those on your medical team, you will likely have to get personal quickly. I still chuckle at the first appointment with my oncologist; both my parents were in attendance and I had just met this doctor. While we hit it off right away, he had to do a physical exam to make notes of what he felt on my body for swollen lymph nodes. Without going into too much detail that would make you laugh and embarrass me, lymph nodes are *all over* your body, so my oncologist was suddenly pressing and squeezing pretty much all over me with my parents sitting right there!

As you determine who will be on your team, make sure you are asking those questions from the list you have thought about and prepared in advance as I recommend in the "Twelve Dos and Don'ts at Diagnosis" chapter. Impromptu questions will certainly come up and you should find out how your medical team can speak to those in-between your formal appointments with them. While few will give you their cell or home numbers, you should know how to submit questions and get them responded to in a reasonable period of time.

Ask your team what they are recommending for treatment, what this recommendation is based on (successfully treating how many others, reading research, etc.), what other options there are that they are not recommending for the first approach, and, if you feel inclined, who else you could speak with about treatments. You deserve to feel well-informed on *all* the options out there so you can make a decision as an informed, empowered patient. It is your diagnosis, health, and life.

Speaking to other professionals aside from those with your new medical team, you will likely think of those at work in your job or, if you are an entrepreneur, in your own business. While you will make a list of those you want to tell personally, speaking to people one-by-one is both time-consuming and exhausting (as I found out)! It begins to feel silly repeating yourself over and over (and over) because you are only speaking to one person at a time. Aside from mass e-mail, there are so many ways we all have at our fingertips to notify the masses.

I think it is your individual decision *how* you tell *whom* and *when*. Your diagnosis is your news after all. Do you want to tell people or is it okay if others tell them? You can choose to tell people on a "need-to-know" basis, but realize you often cannot control whom those that you tell decide to tell! No matter how much you do, it is inevitable that people you do not think of who have known you will hear it through the grapevine.

Cancer is quite a piece of gossip, as you probably know from hearing of others before who had cancer. I certainly heard from, can I say, ex-friends who *somehow* heard the news. I heard from old boyfriends; I heard from old boyfriends' wives! In some cases, my diagnosis helped me put past fall-outs in perspective and get back in touch with people I am very happy to have back in my life.

Today anyone can have a blog (I mentioned my CaringBridge page I quickly set-up within seventy-two hours of confirming my diagnosis), YouTube account or way to post videos, Facebook, Twitter, and many other modes of mass communication or social media. I am just listing the ones most people use communicating over the Internet. I sent some mass text messages to people too.

Naturally, I started with telling those who were the closest to me, and then I worked my way out. I did use Facebook status updates, but did not announce it to immediate family that way! Depending on the status of your relationships with some family, that may be how you want them to find out. As I said before, it's your news and your decision. I am not going to tell you in this chapter the only right way to notify people; just that how you notify whom and when is something you need to think about.

Thanks to an old college friend at Facebook, I was able to retrieve my status updates from around my testing and diagnosis phase. I did not think to save them at the time, as I did not know back then I would be writing a book. I was just a newly diagnosed cancer patient just like you. I share some of them quoted exactly, so you can see I too went through the range of emotions that I tell you it is perfectly okay and natural to feel. I just refused to stay there, but moved into handling cancer using humor and the power of positivity, and handling "Cancer with Joy."

March 13, 2010 (9:54 a.m.): "Yesterday was definitely 1 of the WORST Days of My Whole Life. A Dr.'s appt. turned into a VERY unexpected IV & CT scan & this next Thurs. I'm seeing a specialist to 'find out more.' I'm really not prepared to share any details until I know more & can wrap my head around this, but it's a rather freaky time! If you're sending up a prayer & could give me a mention I would Really Appreciate it!!"

March 15, 2010 (10:24 a.m.): "(Joy Huber) has decided since Thurs. afternoon & my appt. w/ a medical specialist to confirm anything for sure will not be here for approx. 76 hours (but who's counting, ha!). I'm going to be in denial for the next few days. It's not a bad place to be sometimes…I'll keep you posted, and if you read this & go, "What?" just check my page for previous status. Thanks for all your prayers & kind words! I Really Appreciate them!"

March 25, 2010 (10:11 a.m.): "Did get a Cancer diagnosis confirmed yesterday afternoon. Lymphoma. I do not know yet what it is as I see the oncologist tomorrow to, say it with me, 'find out more.' My hunch is they'll do some tests, and I will, WAIT, to find out specifics. If you can't tell, my strategy through this will be lots of Laughter & Humor through the many tears that will fall. I appreciate your support!!"

April 13, 2010 (9:37 a.m.): "(Joy Huber) starts my 1st round of chemo tomorrow. I'll admit anxiety because it's a big dose that will take the ENTIRE day to administer…we're talkin' 8 hours. I don't know how my body will react & what side effects there will be yet—eek!! I appreciate any encouraging words as I enter 'treatment phase' & the battle begins to really rage inside my body. Thanks!"

I share these few examples with you so you can read directly what I said and exactly how I shared with the masses on Facebook. You notice I tried to ward off all the questions in comments when I did not know any more information. I shared my initial feelings of being scared (freaked out!), in denial, and having anxiety ahead of chemo. They are all very natural and you may feel them too. I just do not want you to stay in those places where those emotions are *all* you are feeling. I want to help you find ways to have cancer and be happy—to handle it with joy!

I tried to have face-to-face conversations if someone was geographically close or at least over the telephone with those I was emotionally closest to at the time. Only you know who is on your friends list on Facebook. Are they all personal friends or do you have business contacts intermingled? (I have a personal account, and then business pages set-up for both Joy Huber Presentations, Inc., my company, and now "Cancer with Joy" the brand. If you are on Facebook, *Like* "Cancer with Joy" to be plugged in to the latest!) If you are Facebooking and Tweeting about your tests before anything is confirmed, then potentially all of your friends and followers could find out before your grandma who has never used a computer! It's something to think about.

If you are employed at diagnosis, you can potentially visit confidentially with human resources or consult your employee handbook for tips or policies. Larger companies normally offer as a benefit EAPs, or employee assistance programs, so remember that is a potential resource for you to utilize.

As a business communications expert who has delivered many keynotes and trainings about communication skills, I recommend telling your boss, and the closest work contacts face-to-face if possible. Face-to-face communication makes it possible for people to not only hear our words and our tone or how we say them, but they receive the meaning of the message from our body language and facial expressions as well.

I know those who felt they would be too emotional sharing the news at work in-person so they opted to send an e-mail. Remember with e-mail, the body language and facial expressions are certainly gone, and the tone inferred would be based on how well the recipients know you and whether they can "hear" how you would say those words. With e-mail, choose the most specific words possible versus generic sentences like, "I'm really doing just fine with all of this." Are you *really* just fine and is that said with a sincere tone? Or is your tone sarcastic?

In the official resources chapter, I will share more resources on communicating the news and managing relationships from your diagnosis through treatment. I do want to tell you now about a resource called, "Questions and Answers About Cancer in the Workplace and the Americans with Disabilities Act (ADA)," available at www.eeoc.gov/facts/cancer.html.

Regarding other ways to announce the news of your diagnosis, I am familiar with examples where people announced using a video message posted to a blog and then e-mailed people the link. They did this to communicate face-to-face but avoid having to deal with all the immediate responses (verbal and non-verbal) and questions. You think kids say the darndest things?

When sharing your diagnosis, the things people say and do will be about as diverse as the people you are speaking with, I assure you. Of course, what any of us knows or thinks about a given subject (including cancer) is a culmination of all our previous knowledge and experiences. If you said the word *tornado* to me, I will have a different response than someone else you say this word to based on my experience growing up in Kansas.

People will ask obvious questions, like, "Are you scared?"

"YES, of COURSE I'm scared."

If and how you want to maintain the relationship with them will dictate your response! Many will tell you stories of someone they have known who battled cancer and lost. I wish I knew *why* people choose to tell you these things right at this moment, but they do. You will also hear stories of someone they know who battled cancer and is doing fine today. Remember they are just taking the word *cancer*, and in their mind they are associating it with whatever other knowledge or experience they have on the subject. Most do not know what to say, so the most inappropriate thing they may well regret saying later could come out. Try to be forgiving. Cancer is definitely an uncomfortable subject.

One thing I am thankful I thought to do when sharing my news with people was letting them know how best to follow-up with me, and how I would keep them informed. A cancer diagnosis is the beginning of a long road and naturally people are curious for updates. They likely do not realize how overwhelming it is trying to respond to so many concerned people at once. While I was very grateful for everyone I heard from right at my initial diagnosis, I was also overwhelmed and stressed feeling like I had so many to respond to, call back, e-mail, text, etc. I notice in particular on Facebook, some friends do not seem to acknowledge good news by commenting, but comment on my bad news so quickly. I think it goes back to why we slow down and stare when passing an accident on the road.

As I began my treatment, my Facebook status updates directed people to my CaringBridge site to keep up on the latest versus trying to respond individually to all the comments and messages. I communicated up-front I would *not* be able to respond individually until things calmed down for me. I said how I appreciated everyone understanding that my time and energy would be devoted to attending frequent medical appointments and dealing with the side effects of my treatment including cancer-related fatigue (CRF). I believe if you communicate that message consistently, people will get it and understand. Do not feel overwhelmed; when you catch up with them eventually, you can apologize if you feel the need, but they know you have cancer and most will not need an apology considering the circumstances.

One thing to remember regarding your professional and personal relationships is as your treatment begins and wears on, all the people you initially heard from will *not* constantly be in contact. There will be days you find yourself proactively reaching out in your relationships versus reactively responding because the phone is not ringing, etc. As you know from your pre-cancer life, everyone is busy. Some people sent me one get-well card possibly thinking (I cannot speak for what someone else thinks), "Yes, Joy has cancer. Well, I *sent* a card. Check off the list; that's taken care of. Now…what else? Oh, yes, we need a loaf of bread at the store."

The old cliché you find out who your friends are is definitely true! It can be such a blessing to find out who is really there for you when you need them. You will be disappointed by people you would have sworn would be there for you, and they are not. But you find out and it is always good to know. I have a phrase I use (I actually learned it from an old boyfriend of mine). I say, "Duly noted." My mom laughs when I say this; it is my way of saying I can certainly forgive people, but I will likely not forget. It will be hard for me to drop everything I have going to rush to the side of someone who I thought would be there for me but was not!

I believe relationships are all about two-way communication and feedback to stay healthy. If someone is not offering the communication or behavior you expect of them, what's wrong with giving them feedback that your needs are not being met? Choose your battles carefully during this time but you could certainly communicate a message to the effect of,

> I feel disappointed and saddened. When you said, "let me know what you need," I felt you would be more responsive in helping me out. I want to share I have not felt very supported in my fight against <insert your cancer here>. I have felt alone. I understand you are extremely busy, but I wanted to talk to you about my feelings, and see if you would be willing to make a commitment to help out with <insert specific thing you are seeking assistance with here: picking up groceries, helping with laundry, coming over to visit regularly if you cannot get out to play golf with them or meet up like you used to>.

For the most part, I put my energy and time towards positive thinking, finding humor, handling "Cancer with Joy," and did not have the aforementioned conversation with people. I have found most people take their cues from you reacting in a way similar to how you are handling cancer, since it is after all happening to *you*. When I handled it with joy and demonstrated that through my positivity, attitude, and jokes, most people took it very well. There are those who mistakenly perhaps made offensive cracks (I will give them the benefit of the doubt and say it was likely out of awkwardness and not knowing what to say). I knew I picked my response to those comments, and I chose to let them roll off my back and not impact me for long.

I had enough to battle and someone's passing comment was not going to bring me down. I mainly observed what people said and did, and was occasionally disappointed, but mostly delighted in the wonderful circle of people I have made sure to surround myself with. For anyone who disappointed me there were probably two who pleasantly surprised me by stepping up. There truly are angels among us!

For many of you reading this as a caregiver, family member, or friend of the newly diagnosed, I will go further in the caregivers chapter into how you can be a friend to someone with cancer, and discuss what to say and do. (Caregivers can share these tips and direct others by having conversations with them perhaps before they see the cancer patient.) My final point here is that many of us know the "golden rule," which says "Treat others like *you* want to be treated." What if you switched that up and treated others the way *they* want to be treated? While you may think you would want one thing if you were the one diagnosed and in treatment, your friend possibly prefers something different than what you are thinking.

If you do not know how to treat them, ask what they would prefer. As a cancer patient, I always appreciate it when people acknowledge all I have been through (because cancer is a big part of my life), but then treated me quite normally like before (because cancer is not my whole life and I still want to talk about other things).

While virtually everyone made the comments, "You don't look sick!" to me or I frequently heard, "You look great!" (Thanks! I think? I wanted to be acknowledged for all that I was going through, and then told I looked great. Not told I looked great in a way that seemed to say in tone, "Oh, you must not be going through *too* much. You look fine. You *look* normal." Well, I am trying unbelievably hard to *look normal.* I did not want to look obviously sick and invite stares people seem to not be able to help!)

I want to delve deeper into some relationship circumstances you may have that I have real personal experience with during my time of diagnosis and treatment. While not the easiest to publicly discuss, my goal here is sharing with you to help you, regardless of my personal comfort! The first is that of intimate relationships. As I mentioned, when I was initially diagnosed I was single but ironically re-connecting with an old boyfriend. While it was great that he knew me pre-cancer, his memories of me were always with shoulder-length hair or chin-length at the shortest but certainly not bald! There were physical changes in me throughout my treatment that he had to adjust to.

On our first date in May 2010, I was wearing a halo (ring of hair with a bald spot for the majority of my head since it was nearly Memorial Day weekend and warm) with a cute hat over it (obviously covering the bald spot). I am sure I joked with him about it, but I let him know this was not my real hair, since it looked very much like my old style, length, and color. It made me comfortable to look like *me*, and possibly reassured him to see I did not look drastically different. Come to think of it, I had posted pictures on Facebook (where he's a friend) of me with my short hair when we cut it, so when he saw my shoulder-length hair he probably knew it was fake. I certainly had visions of him trying to run his fingers through my hair and it moving. Uncomfortable! But at the same time I would have just laughed!

I am not sure I would have gone on dates with "new guys" during this time. Remember at diagnosis I had a plan in motion to move away to Nashville, so I was thrilled to be single and be able to go for my dream without trying to convince someone moving should be part of their dream too. I now believe for the right person who truly wants to be with me, since being in Nashville is my dream, it will be part of theirs too to be with me, and they will be thrilled in my pursuit of it!

On our "first date back together," I was so touched to sit down at Hu-Hot Mongolian Grill with my plate and realize a small jewelry box was on the table pushed over to my side! Remember, I have known this guy since my twenty-first birthday in 1997. He had alluded to having made jewelry purchases for me when we had previously dated that he never gave me because we had broken up. While I was a little nervous since this box was the size of a ring box, I knew this guy well enough to know his practical side. I was certainly not being proposed to on our "first date back together" at Hu-Hot.

When I opened it, there was a beautiful pair of heart-shaped diamond earrings that I had to put on immediately of course! It was a really sweet night and definitely the beginning of something special. I was blessed to feel so comfortable with this guy since he has known me for years and years and knows *me* versus just getting to know me with cancer. That was on a Friday night.

That Saturday I saw my maternal grandparents. I referenced my paternal grandfather before who passed of lung cancer in the 80s. My dad's mom passed in 2005. My maternal grandparents were both relatively healthy and at home. What I did not know then was that Saturday would be the last time I saw my grandpa, who I am extremely close to, alive.

I had my third chemo treatment scheduled for the next Friday. Tuesday afternoon the phone calls started coming in from an uncle and aunt. My eighty-six-year-old (hard-working, independent) grandpa had been in an accident. He was on a tractor with no enclosed cab driving down a highway. When he went to turn onto a side road, a vehicle coming over the hill hit the tractor. He came off the tractor and hit the pavement. He was flown to a trauma center in Lincoln, Nebraska, and when my mom and I arrived we, along with some other family members who were gathered, met with a doctor who told us he had passed about twenty-five minutes earlier.

We eventually went from the hospital to my grandparent's house about two hours away. It was weird having been there a little over three days before, when he and I ate fruit and white cake while we visited. He was relatively healthy, healthy enough to live at home. By the next Tuesday night, all the kids and grandkids were gathering to prepare for his funeral.

We stayed overnight with my grandma and when I awoke Wednesday morning and realized what had really happened the day before, where I was, and why I was there, hot stinging tears shot out of my eyes and rolled across my face. When I got up, my grandma and mom were writing the obituary (at the same table where we had cake the Saturday afternoon before), and we were planning to go to the mortuary to plan the funeral service.

As we planned the service, I had many wonderful memories to share. I am blessed to have lived driving distance from my grandparents my whole life, and that was one of the things that made me pause on my path straight to Nashville. I have always gotten along well with my grandparents, but as I started my business in late 2005, and was working incredibly hard building it (*lots* of work with no pay!), I became even closer to my grandpa, a fellow entrepreneur as he had started his own rock hauling company and was a farmer. He was a World War II Veteran and was awarded the Purple Heart among many other medals for his service. He was in the U.S. Army on the front lines as a sharpshooter, wounded in battle, and honorably discharged.

But, for me, not knowing a lot about his service over thirty years before I was born, he was "Grandpa." I was the second born of his eight grandchildren. He was someone I wanted to spend time with and truly loved spending time with, not someone you "should" visit as a grandparent. We could sit and visit for hours easily.

He taught me so much through showing more than merely telling. I learned from him that being kind to everyone is the right thing to do (and it feels good too). I learned to treat everyone with respect, because we are all people whether you are a janitor mopping the floor or the CEO, everyone has ideas and dreams. I learned from him faith and positive thinking, hard work, and persistence.

Fortunately, much of the last "normal" day of my life before I confirmed my cancer diagnosis was spent with him. I had a speaking engagement at my former college that evening, and my grandparents live about forty-five minutes from where I was speaking. I went to spend the afternoon visiting with my grandparents while I was in the area. My grandma was gone to play cards, and it was just me and Grandpa. I can still see in my mind where I sat on the couch in the living room and he was in "his chair." We laughed that day, but we talked seriousness too. He could see and knew about the lump in my neck, and by March 23, I had my CT scan, had been sent to Dr. Arrogant, and had the ultrasound needle biopsy. We were just waiting on the results, which came in the next afternoon.

I spoke at the college that night and drove home. The next day, my life changed forever, and it will never be quite the same. Grandpa knew I had cancer when he passed. We had cut my hair at the end of April, and my grandparents came to my parents' to stay a weekend the first of May. Fortunately, we spent that weekend just a few weeks before he passed, hanging out. He nicknamed me "munchy" because I was always munching, eating small snacks throughout the day versus big meals (more on that strategy later). He saw my hair when we cut it short, and even saw me in May with my bald head and some of my various wig looks.

While my family was finalizing funeral arrangements, I was on the phone with my oncologist to get chemo changed. I knew I could not go straight from chemo Friday to visitation that evening, and the funeral was lining up to be Saturday, May 29, the Saturday kicking off Memorial Day Weekend. I managed to get my chemo moved to Thursday. After picking out flowers, we drove approximately two hours home. I had chemo number three Thursday, Friday we went to the hospital to get my Neulasta® shot the day after chemo, and then we headed for the visitation that evening. The funeral was Saturday.

The spot of Grandpa's accident is just down the road (walking distance) from my grandparent's house. I frequently have to drive by the spot either going to or coming from their place, which is incredibly difficult. The tears shoot from my eyes uncontrollably, and I am fine with that. If I had not loved so deeply, I would not feel such a sense of loss.

My boyfriend at the time met me outside the funeral. This was essentially our second date. His mom also attended. I was incredibly grateful he could be there with me, as I definitely gripped his hand when the twenty-one-gun salute for military was fired. I was standing at the burial service at the cemetery, not too far behind my grandma, and I remember when the folded flag was presented to her. "This flag is given to you on behalf of a grateful nation . . ." is about all I remember before dissolving in tears. It was definitely nice to have someone who had known me about thirteen years, and my family on that side, around then.

With two hours between where we each were living at the time, it became necessary to spend long weekends together. He worked Monday-Friday and sometimes on the weekend with his job. It made sense for me to go to his place since my business was suspended while I was going through chemo once every three weeks. I distinctly remember how nervous I was the first of those weekends.

At this point, we had shaved my head and I was bald. While he knew this, he had not seen my bald head and I was not sure I wanted him to. I recall struggling with, "Would he be attracted to me? ME? Minus my hair?!" I kept thinking of the country song sung by Randy Travis, "Forever and Ever Amen." There is a line in there that says, "Honey, I don't care, I ain't in love with your hair, and if it all fell out, I'd love you anyways." Well, we were about to find out!

I remember the first weekend we were planning for me to stay there and stay overnight. I asked him if he had a guest bedroom I could sleep in. His response was basically, "Don't be silly!" I was quite terrified of us trying to sleep in and the sunlight streaming in through his windows lighting up my bald head lying in bed next to him! I also knew I was not going to sleep in a wig (uncomfortable) just to "wake up with hair."

In handling "Cancer with Joy" fashion, I thought, *How could we make this fun?* I remembered how much fun I had doing my online fashion show and trying on different looks. I would take different "hair looks," short wigs, longer wigs, hats, etc., to his place for my visits. I did not *have* to have the same hair every day so why not mix it up? A friend of his would be over one day and I would have my long hair wig on. The same friend would come over the very next day and I would have a short hair wig on. They would just smile! I made it fun, switching from long hair to short back to long effortlessly!

I must say my boyfriend also went with the changes well, but I know I would not have continued to date someone who did not. You want people who truly love you for *you* around during your treatment and battle. If someone only loves you with a certain hairstyle, and is not understanding of your changing looks during this time, then I encourage you to focus on surrounding yourself with people who care about the person you are internally and are not concerned with if you have short hair, long hair, no hair, etc.

When a bunch of wigs came in the mail, I tried them on for him and got his opinion on what he liked and didn't. As my hair grew back, we would joke about who had longer hair—him or me. I was the same person internally he cared for, and I guess that's what mattered for him! Everyone's appearance changes over time anyways; if he teased me about not looking the same as when I met him on my twenty-first birthday, I would give it right back, and say, "Neither do you!" By Christmas, he gave me a beautiful pearl ring with diamond accents! He also gave me thoughtful gifts like a baseball cap from his workplace (I was needing more hats for variety), and a hooded sweatshirt if I wanted to cover my then-becoming-fuzzy head by just throwing a hood up to keep warm.

I have had many people ask me about dating and intimate relationships during cancer treatment. I know from my personal experience it is all definitely possible. If you are married or in a relationship, I would say the best thing to do is talk openly and honestly with your spouse or partner about the changes and how they make you feel. It is hard for them to know what you are thinking or what you need unless you tell them; this is likely uncharted territory for them too.

If you are single, I think the decision on whether to pursue a relationship or not at this time is up to you. I have always been a very independent woman who is happier single than dating the wrong person. I definitely do not have to be dating someone. I rather enjoy being single and find my thoughts, or a book I am immersed in, interesting enough company at dinner for one. I was single by choice at my diagnosis; since I was preparing to move, I was not interested in starting to date someone. Then what? A long-distance relationship is an option, and many successfully juggle this.

I believe if I were single and interested in meeting and/or dating someone while going through treatment, I would have looked for someone else going through cancer treatment or who was a survivor having been through it. I believe support groups are wonderful places to meet new people who have gone through or are going through what you are, and that is a good community in which to make new contacts that could develop into genuine friendships and even more romantically.

I have also been asked many questions about relationships with children and cancer so I want to touch on that here. There will be more about this in the resources chapter and as part of your bonus in the back of the book! I have no children, so the first thing I want to address is the fertility consideration. It was exactly three weeks from my diagnosis to my first chemo treatment, and many other things were happening. I do not recall having a conversation with anyone though on my medical team or in my family about fertility. That is why I mention it to make sure it is a consideration of yours, at least between diagnosis and treatment. There is a great article at Cancer.org titled, "Preserving Fertility in Women" (www.cancer.org/treatment/treatmentsandsideeffects/physicalsideeffects/fertilityandcancerwhataremyoptions/fertility-and-cancer-preserving-fertility-in-women).

There is also an article on preserving fertility in men at www.cancer.org/treatment/treatmentsandsideeffects/physicalsideeffects/fertilityandcancerwhataremyoptions/fertility-and-cancer-preserving-fertility-in-men.

A story from a personal friend of mine, contributor Cristy Norwood, on how she handled "Cancer with Joy" in chapter three shares her experience of being pregnant when she was diagnosed with breast cancer. I want to share about telling children of your diagnosis too. My closest personal experience with going through treatment with a child around comes from my only nephew who was just over six when I was diagnosed. I did not have to tell him personally of my diagnosis though.

The American Cancer Society has an entire resource section on this online. I located a terrific article titled, "Helping Children When a Family Member Has Cancer: Dealing With Diagnosis." This comprehensive section is at www.cancer.org/treatment/childrenandcancer/helpingchildrenwhenafamilymemberhascancer. Much like I mentioned before on open, honest communication with your partner if you are in a relationship, I believe the same should be done with children (considering their age, of course, for what is appropriate).

Please make sure you read through the resources chapter for many wonderful additional resources that will be helpful to you in handling your relationships as you move from initial diagnosis into cancer treatment. Obviously your diagnosis has caused changes in your life, and it will impact all of your relationships. My cancer diagnosis definitely caused some interesting things to happen in my relationships; everyone will react differently and some things will disappoint you while others pleasantly surprise you. I know people take their cues from you, so when you move beyond the initial normal and understandable but possibly negative emotions to mainly facing "Cancer with Joy," that gives children and others a sense of calm and helps relationships.

Chapter Seven
Emotional &
Physical Fitness

One of my goals with my "Cancer with Joy" brand and this first book to come from the brand is to give you the essential resource at diagnosis. Many of these topics can be covered in more depth, but I want you to have one book you (and those on your team) can read that provides initial valuable information. I want to save you time, money, and precious energy. I want to tell you some of my stories (and share stories from others) of handling "Cancer with Joy" to inspire you to handle your own diagnosis and treatment using humor and the power of positivity!

Cancer is an emotional ride though; I know that well! The number two "do" I shared with you at diagnosis is "do" get mad, sad, bitter, depressed, etc. Then I encourage you not to stay there throughout your journey! I wanted to add to what is already in this book by giving you some additional food for your emotional soul! That's part of what this chapter is about! I also want to talk about physical activity and share some nutrition information. I am a firm believer in what you eat and how much activity you get will no doubt impact how you feel emotionally!

The website *www.dictionary.com* defines nutrition as "The process by which living organisms obtain food and use it for growth, metabolism, and repair. The stages of nutrition include ingestion, digestion, absorption, transport, assimilation, and excretion." I list in the resources chapter several very good websites that talk about cancer, cooking, and nutrition. There is also an exceptional book called *What to Eat During Cancer Treatment: 100 Great-Tasting, Family-Friendly Recipes to Help You Cope*, published by the American Cancer Society.

First, nausea is a cancer and related treatment side effect I believe a majority of people have. I personally was not throwing up a lot in the days following chemo, but what I experienced was a *feeling* of sickness. I think today you do not have to accept that this is just part of your treatment and the cancer battle. Continue to dialogue with those on your medical team about this and continue to try different things. I found it very helpful to keep a log of what I ate and how I felt.

My oncologists' office told me to have something light before chemotherapy. Ask your medical team what you can have before and throughout the entire course of treatment. I was very into snacking my way through cancer treatment; remember that my grandpa nicknamed me "munchy" because I was always munching? With my fear of getting sick, I would eat something little and see how it went. When it stayed down fine, I would munch on something else little. Some snacks that personally worked well for me included: a hard-boiled egg, sliced apple and peanut butter, packages of cheese and crackers, a scoop of cottage cheese with sliced peaches, applesauce, milkshakes, and toast with cinnamon sugar. These all incorporate protein, fruits, dairy, and breads.

I got more into juicing than I had before diagnosis. I bought my first juicer and the fresh juice tasted so wonderful! When I want a treat and don't want to clean up the juicer (or figure out what to do with the dehydrated pulp), I greatly enjoy fresh carrot-apple juice at Juice Stop.

I firmly believe that battling "Cancer with Joy" is a culmination of what you eat and good nutrition, adjusted by how you are feeling to manage the treatment side effects, married to staying physically active, so let's discuss physical activity next.

The National Cancer Institute's Fact Sheet defines physical activity as "any bodily movement produced by skeletal muscles; such movement results in an expenditure of energy. Physical activity is a critical component of energy balance, a term used to describe how weight, diet, and physical activity influence health, including cancer risk" (see www.cancer.gov/cancertopics/factsheet/prevention/physicalactivity). Regarding how much physical activity adults need, the website says, "the Centers for Disease Control and Prevention (CDC) recommend that adults 'engage in moderate-intensity physical activity for at least 30 minutes on five or more days of the week' or 'engage in vigorous-intensity physical activity for at least 20 minutes on three or more days of the week.'" That is not considering cancer and your specific treatment plan.

The short answer, of course, is to talk with your medical team about how much physical activity you have been getting, and what you plan to try to do to get their approval, thoughts, concerns, and suggestions. The year before I was diagnosed with stage four cancer, I had my fifteen-year high school class reunion! Like most people getting ready for a class reunion, I decided to up the physical activity to see if it would be possible to "lose a few extra pounds" before going back. I have always enjoyed riding a bike, and got on the exercise bike more regularly.

I enjoy getting out and riding my bike and taking in the fresh air. One of the persistent big side effects of my chemo treatment, even aside from the cancer-related fatigue, that makes me not want to bike for twenty-five minutes at a time, has been dry mouth. I have even tried and successfully used new products specifically for it including toothpastes, mouthwashes, sprays, and gum. I definitely drink more water now than before and have successfully kicked my former regular need for sweet soft drinks! I will admit to having an occasional soda every now and then but I used to drink approximately two cans of pop almost every day.

With my mouth getting so dry, vigorously pedaling the exercise bike wasn't the ideal option while in chemo treatment. I switched to more walking instead; unfortunately I have never been a runner.

I would encourage you to consider three things when it comes to physical activity in cancer treatment: 1) have a conversation about it with those on your medical team who have your vitals, know your diagnosis and the treatment you are receiving, and are seeing you physically and conducting regular tests and exams; 2) incorporate what you can based on how you feel into your schedule; and 3) listen to your body and what it is telling you. There were days I was feeling good and thought I could probably walk further out in one direction, but then I remembered I had to turn around and walk all the way back home. I decided not to push it considering how recently I had received chemo, and realized the activity I had gotten was better than nothing at all! The Cancer Society offers more information at www.cancer.org/treatment/ survivorshipduringandaftertreatment/stayingactive/physical-activity-and-the-cancer-patient.

For the most part, trying to incorporate some physical activity into my regular routine helped me feel better overall, including thinking positive and feeling positive emotions. We all have good and bad days, and I have not handled "Cancer with Joy" every single day! On the day I consider the most physically painful, when the stent that was in my right kidney was removed, I still tried to face that procedure using humor. I was cracking jokes about jumping out at an intersection close to my urologists' office and running the opposite direction down the street! See, the closer we got to the office and going in, of course the more anxiety I felt!

On the days when I felt negative emotions creeping in, I thought, *I don't want to waste precious time feeling negative about this.* I wondered if there was some emotional food I could snack on that would help inspire me. Fortunately, there is! I hope you consider this book a big part of inspiring you on ways to handle "Cancer with Joy" most of the time! Aside from the chapters presenting my story, the ten (+ a bonus) ways I handled "Cancer with Joy," and the ten stories (eleven—there is also a bonus story in that chapter if you counted!) from others, here are some *more* things for you to read, listen to, and consider.

Many people simply have a fear of the unknown. Ask yourself if learning more about your cancer, the treatment your medical team is recommending, etc., will help you feel better. This is why I suggest at the first "do" that you "do" get a second opinion and that you "do" go to someone who makes you comfortable! Talk to more than just one medical professional about your diagnosis and treatment. Going to UNMC and having a second professional agree on my treatment plan helped ease a lot of the negative emotions I possibly would have felt for a prolonged period of time if I had not gotten the second professional to weigh in.

This is why I also suggest early on that you "don't" go to the Internet as your primary initial source of information. In the resources chapter, I list some very good sources you or someone on your support team can look up to learn more. There may be times you do not want to know more because it will make you more nervous. I again go to my extreme fear of tornadoes as an example. I grew up in Kansas and have many friends who would go out during a storm and want to see what the clouds were doing and what was happening. I NEVER felt this way (hence my family likes to tell a story about finding me at a young age in the bedroom closet with a blanket thrown over my head during a severe thunderstorm)! I didn't want to see at all what was happening around me!

As mentioned earlier in this book, after I achieved remission, I had an abnormal Pap smear in October 2010, which escalated into cervical biopsies and the need for the LEEP to be done in December 2010. I was on the Internet looking up information about this procedure thinking it would make me feel better and remove the negative emotions by getting informed. Then I had a change of heart.

I decided since I would not be awake and aware during the procedure there was no need to find out everything they would be doing to me! As I have told my dentist, it is amazing what you can do to people when they are numb! Based on the sounds I can hear when at my dentist, I know they are doing some pretty intense things inside my mouth, but, I am numb and do not feel it, so I do not need to see it or know too much about exactly what is happening! That is an individual decision for you to make.

This is why I also recommend as "do" number nine, "do" talk to someone who has "been there." In the resources chapter, there is an entire section listing sources of support and many groups including *Imerman Angels* who will match you up "with someone who has fought and survived the same type of cancer." If you want to speak to me, I enjoy getting to know and working with individuals so much that I went back to school to be professionally trained in coaching. In addition to presenting my "Cancer with Joy" program to groups, I also offer limited individual and small group coaching. You can contact my team to learn more about any of this by completing the form at www.JoyHuber.com/contact or by e-mailing coaching@cancerwithjoy.com.

In addition to the physical activity to help us burn some of the energy our emotions give us, things including reading, writing, and listening (to others or to music) can be helpful in working through the negative emotions so we can feel the positive ones. Read these things and then write about how you are feeling. Do you have a journal? It does not need to be anything fancy; any notebook will work to record your private thoughts. Date these entries; they are always fun to review. A CaringBridge journal or any blog you set up is a public way of journaling, so decide whether you want others to be able to read and comment on your thoughts or if you want to keep them to yourself.

This poem has really helped me. On the days when I feel like cancer is massive, on the days when I would look in the mirror and see all cancer had been able to take from me (most notably my shoulder-length hair!), on the days when I doubted for a second if I could *really* conquer this thing, I would read:

What Cancer Cannot Do

Cancer is so limited…
It cannot cripple Love
It cannot shatter Hope
It cannot corrode Faith
It cannot destroy Peace
It cannot kill Friendship
It cannot suppress Memories
It cannot silence Courage
It cannot invade the Soul
It cannot steal eternal Life
It cannot conquer the Spirit

—Author Unknown

I instantly feel better reading that! I am inspired, I feel brave, I am full of courage, and I *know* I can beat this thing! There is so much cancer cannot do!

Another personal favorite of mine is the "Attitude" poem by Charles Swindoll (excerpt here by permission).

Attitude

The remarkable thing is we have a choice every day regarding the attitude we will embrace for that day… I am convinced that life is 10% what happens to me and 90% how I react to it.

I also previously shared with you the E + R = O formula in Jack Canfield's wonderful book *The Success Principles*. It is not merely the event in our life that dictates the outcome, but our response is factored into that event, and *that* is what ultimately dictates the outcome!

At www.hopegarden.com/cancer.html I discovered this delightful quote attributed to John Diamond: "Cancer is a word, not a sentence."

This quote, by Author Unknown, says, "Some see a hopeless end, while others see an endless hope."

As a songwriter, I find energy in music, and a song can literally turn my day around. I encourage you to visit www.CancerwithJoyBook. com to listen to my two co-written songs "Live Before I Die" (ironically finished before I ever heard the word "cancer" associated with me!) and "Bright Side Effects." If I found "bright side effects" including thinking the paper cuts I got from get well cards were a neat thing, what "bright side effects" can you find on a daily basis while in cancer treatment? Take a blank piece of paper, write "Blessings" at the top, and just start writing. Things as simple as "I have clean water readily available to me to drink," filled me with an immense feeling of gratitude. I did not have hair on my head like most of my friends my age, but an activity like this focuses you on what you have versus what you do not have. It is an amazing activity!

Next up, some tips for your caregivers, and even family and friends.

Chapter Eight
For Caregivers

I believe the essential resource on cancer for the newly diagnosed should include useful information for caregivers. Your caregiver may be one person or a team who takes turns. Even if you enlist one primary caregiver, remember they will need rest and care also to keep from getting burnt out. Being a caregiver to someone newly diagnosed with cancer is an emotional and physically taxing thing.

Being an unmarried young adult, my primary caregiver was definitely my mom. She went with me to the most medical appointments, and frequently held the list of questions we had compiled before the appointment while taking copious notes. She took pictures to help document the journey (you get to see these as part of your bonus with purchasing this book), and dressed up in costume for the appropriate holidays (e.g., the Easter bunny, and sporting flashing reindeer antlers) as we faced "Cancer with Joy." She served as my primary grocery shopper, cook, deliverer of frequent snacks and water on trays, and prescription picker upper!

She also had to give her opinion on many unpleasant things as I experienced them, and helped determine when something was *normal* and when I should alert part of my medical team. Your caregiver should definitely be someone who cares for you deeply and does not mind these things because of their commitment to getting you well. Mom was in the room watching a lot of blood being drawn, IVs being started, and times my port was accessed. She had to inspect everything from blood in the stool (there was a lot after the stent was removed from my kidney, and I needed a second opinion on whether it was normal or too much) to worse. While I realize this is all unpleasant, it is important to know when selecting and accepting the caregiver role.

In the resource chapter, I share a website called *Lotsa Helping Hands.* You can create your community at <u>www.lotsahelpinghands.com/</u> <u>create</u>. I did not find out about this until after my main treatment had concluded. Actually I discovered it, along with so many other time and energy-saving resources, when I was doing all the research for this book. I have taken a lot of time, so you do not have to because you hold this essential resource in your hands. I recommend you take the time to create your community and list what you anticipate needing help with, whether it is delivering a home-cooked meal a few nights a week or doing a couple loads of laundry or giving the cancer patient a ride to a medical appointment so the caregiver does not have to take off from work. So many well-meaning friends and family sincerely want to help and this is a terrific tool to organize them into a community that offers much-needed support to the caregiver.

I located this specific link on *Cancer.org* for you (<u>www.cancer.</u> <u>org/treatment/caregivers/caregiving/whatyouneedtoknow.index</u>).   In the resources chapter, I also devoted a whole section to resources for caregivers, friends, and family. Remember caregivers can also need and receive one-on-one support through organizations including *Imerman Angels* if you need someone to talk to about the additional demands you are juggling!

Helping other family and friends with what to say and do can be a large job for a caregiver. I know from my personal experience that many in the family would tell my parents, "I don't know what to say or do." They felt awkward with me being a young adult with stage four cancer! Fortunately, there are resources that I took the time to locate for you that offer wonderful tips. Caregivers may be teaching these to others or giving helpful hints on what might be most appreciated based on being so close to the cancer patient and knowing more of their thoughts and feelings.

Here is another useful link at *Cancer.org* (www.cancer.org/cancer/ news/features/when-someone-you-know-has-cancer). Regarding dos and don'ts for the person supporting the cancer patient, remember I shared how much I wanted to be acknowledged for my fight rather than having it dismissed because I "looked fine." I talk more about how important it is to be acknowledged later in this chapter. A "don't" that I would share from my personal experience is try not to give the patient information they did not ask for. I personally had this happen several times, likely from those who meant well, but instead I would ask if the patient was interested in hearing or learning more. Please do not push a bunch of reading or go on and on about a treatment or subject they did not ask about or seem interested in!

Also remember earlier I suggested you simply ask the cancer patient how they want to be treated or what they would most appreciate. I would add that you could offer a few different options to let them choose from instead of asking a totally open question like, "What can I do to help?" Try, "I'm planning to do something for you after this week's chemo treatment. Would you prefer me to do your grocery shopping Saturday morning or a few loads of laundry (including the ironing!) Sunday afternoon?"

In the resources chapter, I share a tremendous resource I located called www.circusofcancer.org. It says "a how-to site to help you step right up when your friend has breast cancer." Caregivers can point family and friends towards sites like this or suggest specific things listed that they know the patient would really appreciate. The terrific thing about this site is so much of the advice can also be utilized for any friend or family member battling any kind of cancer.

It suggests upon first hearing the news that you do make contact, but keep it brief. I was a big fan of all the *thinking of you* cards I received with checks in it suggesting I or my caregiver get a treat on the sender. Many sent gift cards; at least take a minute to write a thoughtful, personalized note versus just signing your name! It is very thoughtful if you let the cancer patient know that you know they have a lot going on and they can take their time responding to you. There is a lot going on when you first confirm a diagnosis.

One of the best things a caregiver could remind family and friends to do is be consistent throughout the battle. As I write this book, I am still receiving maintenance chemo treatments. I know when some people heard the word "remission," I was completely forgotten about; some forgot about me after they sent one get-well card! Consistent brief visits, phone calls, cards and e-cards, e-mails, notes on CaringBridge, etc., are so much better than one long phone call asking a million questions and then never inquiring again. As I said in the relationships chapter, I definitely experienced some surprises in my relationships throughout my treatment, but for anyone who disappointed me there were others who pleasantly surprised me.

If you are reading this as a member of a cancer patient's support team, little things mean a lot. Some of these are certainly not little gestures, so you could go together as a group and have each person chip in to create a fund to do something special. Some of my favorite things that people did for me (just to give you some ideas) included: sending me out for a complimentary pedicure; buying me hats when I lost my hair; mailing me from out-of-state a box of goodies after I was bedridden for about a week following the very first chemo that included cozy socks, a soft blanket, and women's magazines; or paying for a Netflix subscription since I had so many days I would just lay around and doze with fatigue and restlessness. My friend Nicole works at a spa and she treated me to a complimentary facial! A friend who had been through cancer and his wife sent me bath goodies to pamper myself. Many friends took me to lunch. Don't forget the caregivers too! You can do things for the cancer patient but taking care of the caregiver helps to ensure good care for the patient!

For the caregiver, while even though at times it can feel like a thankless job, remember you *are* appreciated more than the cancer patient is thinking right now to express (I did not tell you enough, so **THANKS MOM!**). Try not to take negative things the cancer patient expresses too personally, as being right there most of the time will occasionally put you on the receiving end of those negative emotions and thoughts.

No one, caregiver included, should **ever** say to a cancer patient, "I know EXACTLY how you feel"! I very rarely get upset, but this is one thing that inflamed me greatly! Another one that set me off was, "If I were you, this is what I would do." I ignored that, and did not spend as much time with people who would think to even say that! I do not think anyone can say with certainty what they would do if they were in your shoes, and they are not you and are not experiencing exactly what you are, so just do not think to go there! Do not even compare the cancer patient to another person you know who had cancer, or even had the same kind of cancer. "Well, so-and-so had breast cancer too, and this worked for her." Most people do not have all the details of your specific case, plus each cancer patient has a different experience because they are a different person!

Caregivers can use empathy, which to me is **discussing** the emotions that people around them, cancer patient included, are expressing, *without reacting* to them. What I mean by this is if the cancer patient seems frustrated, instead of reacting by saying, "Don't take your frustration out on me!" a much more useful continuation to the conversation would be, "It seems like you are very frustrated. Tell me more about that." This helps the frustrated person calm down because they feel **acknowledged** and understood. Try to be patient and let the patient vent.

Have you ever noticed how when you're waiting for customer service and you haven't been acknowledged you'll clear your throat, say, "Excuse me," or do things just to get attention? Then once the customer service rep. says, "Sorry for the delay; I'll be right with you," you may respond (as I frequently do) by saying, "Oh, no problem!" Do you know *why* it is not a problem anymore? Because you have been acknowledged! This skill goes a <u>long</u> way in caregiving.

Remember to take care of yourself too, and do not be afraid to enlist backup. Do not try to do everything you have been doing previously plus taking on all the additional responsibilities of caregiving. Depending on the patient you are supporting, you will figure out how much help you need. My mom did not even request it, but I know she was very grateful when a next-door neighbor brought over pans of frozen meat/pasta entrees we could just pop in the oven! She also delivered pans of a delicious chocolate dessert that was quite a treat! I was grateful too; this was thoughtful and delicious!

If you need support in the form of someone to talk to, someone who has been there or is a caregiver right now, remember that is all part of the many resources I share in the next chapter. Being a caregiver is usually a volunteer position, but as Lt. Col. James H. Doolittle said, "There's nothing stronger than the heart of a volunteer."

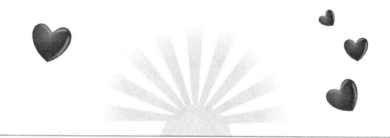

Chapter Nine

Resources You Need to Know About (at Diagnosis)

If you haven't already peeked ahead, after this chapter is the end (of this book). As I have said before though, for you and me, it is really just the beginning. I will be providing you with ongoing support throughout your treatment and beyond. Information on the big bonus is next, and part of that bonus includes updated links and additional resources at www.CancerwithJoyBook.com.

Yes, **updated** links, that is right! I, like you, have bought books and excitedly read about links to resources only to type the address in and find it is broken or no longer takes me where I thought it would go. I wanted to make the commitment that as long as you are a member of the "Cancer with Joy" community at www.CancerwithJoyBook.com I will make the commitment to keep the links to resources up-to-date and make the additional commitment to even *add* to the list.

I will save you precious time and energy finding additional resources, and all you need to do is join www.CancerwithJoyBook.com for the latest! If something is quoted, I of course found it directly on the website I am pointing you towards. There may be variances in the style of content on these websites I am quoting from and how the content in the rest of the book looks. I also want to share that some websites, like www.cancer.org, are so massive and have so much terrific information I found them almost a little overwhelming to the newly diagnosed. Therefore, I am sharing specific links to pages. I may have several resources that are www.cancer.org + pointing to a specific page, but I would rather offer that than just give you www.cancer.org and leave you to take your valuable time trying to wade through it all alone.

More Great Websites from "Cancer with Joy"

www.CancerwithJoyBook.com—This is your first stop to claim your bonus with purchasing this book. Get signed up so you can utilize all the benefits here that help you have cancer *and* be happy! This website features many of my personal photos from my journey, personal video including video from the day we shaved my head, music (this is where you can listen to my co-written song "Bright Side Effects"), and recipes. You can also read information on my LIVE appearances and events (and receive special discounts for members ONLY)! This is *the* website for updates to my story, and to my store where you can get "Cancer with Joy" merchandise including T-shirts and other items. I will *also* share cancer news here, and more stories contributed by others on how they too learned to handle "Cancer with Joy" (to have yours considered to be featured, e-mail stories@cancerwithjoybook.com for guidelines). Don't forget this is also the place to find updated links to resources mentioned here and additional resources we've discovered.

www.cancerwithjoycruise.com—This is your opportunity to take a vacation *with me!* Several times a year (departing from both the east and west coasts), I will be taking cancer patients (with your doctor's written permission), survivors, caregivers, family, and friends on a well-deserved break from the cancer world we have been involuntarily immersed in. This exciting event is limited to only 100 people at a time and fills up **very quickly**, so sign-up and don't delay if you want to go on one this year. On the days at sea we have fun with events (for patients and survivors, and separate ones for caregivers, family, and friends) so you can connect with one another while learning to handle "Cancer with Joy" (literally *with me* LIVE!). On the days in port we take a vacation! What could be more fun?

www.CancerwithJoy.com —"'Cancer with Joy' is FREE! Sign-Up for INSTANT access to: helpful resources, support, en'courage'ment, video of Joy speaking, and information on how to book Joy of 'Cancer with Joy' as a speaker." This is MY FREE website, so if you are not signed up here, please make sure you do that! There are a couple dozen posts here with additional information including cancer news *not* found in this book. There is video of me speaking to a conference for women here. This is where you can also order your own "Cancer with Joy" T-shirt in your choice of the color: pink, turquoise, or grey!

www.Facebook.com/joyfulcommunications#!/pages/Cancer-with-Joy/103382816401554 — The "Cancer with Joy" Facebook page. You can also search "Cancer with Joy" on Facebook to locate us.

www.Twitter.com/cancerwithjoy — Follow "Cancer with Joy" on Twitter.

Cancer Information

---

www.health.usnews.com/best-hospitals/rankings/cancer—"Nearly 900 hospitals are listed in Cancer. All are experienced in treating difficult cases—a hospital is listed only if at least 270 inpatients who needed a high level of expertise in this specialty were treated there in 2006, 2007, and 2008, or if surveyed specialists recommended the hospital for such patients. The top 50 hospitals are ranked by score. Those below the top 50 are listed alphabetically."

www.cancer101.org—"CANCER101's mission is to help patients and caregivers get organized and informed to fight their cancer. They provide CANCER101 Planners to cancer centers in all 50 states to give to their patients and caregivers in need. The planners are free to their patients and include essential organizational tools and important resources designed to empower patients and caregivers to take control over their diagnosis from the moment they learn they have cancer through the next ten years of follow-up care. The planners encourage patients to partner with their medical team: questions are asked and answered, notes and appointments are written down in one place, and patients and caregivers feel in control. And just as importantly, the planner gives patients and their loved ones hope. CANCER101 Now Supports People with Any Cancer."

www.cancer.net—"Oncologist-approved cancer information from the American Society of Clinical Oncology" LOVE it!

www.cancer.about.com—"With more than 800 topic sites (Guide sites), About.com helps users find solutions to a wide range of daily needs—from parenting, health care and technology to cooking, travel and many others." I reference a page from this website in chapter one.

www.empowher.com—"EmpowHER is an award-winning health media company for women. The company's website provides visitors access to one of the largest women's health and wellness content libraries on the web, as well as the largest online community of women discussing their health and wellness issues. EmpowHER promotes a '24 Hour Promise' to its visitors, who can come to the site, ask any health question and receive a response within 24 hours."

www.copingmag.com/cwc—This takes you specifically to the Coping® with Cancer section of copingmag.com. They also offer a magazine and website on Coping® with Allergies & Asthma. "For 25 years, *Coping* has been a source of knowledge, hope, and inspiration to people worldwide. When you need positive and helpful information that relates to a specific medical condition, *Coping* can help:

"Coping® with Cancer Website. The *Coping with Cancer* website is a complete online experience that educates and inspires. It is presented in a warm and friendly, easy-to-use format, and provides information by specific cancer type, general knowledge about living with cancer, and wellness and inspirational topics. The *Coping* media team is constantly adding relevant articles and trustworthy resources.

"Coping® with Cancer magazine is written by and for the cancer community with help from our editors. A wide variety of professionals share their knowledge and experience in easy-to-read, relevant articles, and patients, caregivers, and survivors share their strategies for coping. Add in the latest news, FDA updates, resource lists, and exclusive interviews with celebrity cancer survivors, and the result is a publication that provides a unique editorial environment."

www.awomanshealth.com—This is the website for "Women" magazine and tells you how you can subscribe if you are interested in receiving a magazine focused on "health, wellness, prevention, treatment, community, and cancer."

www.consumerreportshealth.org—"Get expert, unbiased, and fact-based health information from Consumer Reports Health." This website includes sections on: healthy living, conditions and treatments, prescription drugs, natural health, doctors and hospitals, and insurance.

www.cancer.org/acs/groups/content/@editorial/documents/document/acspc-026864.pdf

www.cancer.org/treatment/treatmentsandsideeffects/emotionalsideeffects/index

www.cancer.org/treatment/treatmentsandsideeffects/
physicalsideeffects/index

www.cancer.org/treatment/treatmentsandsideeffects/
complementaryandalternativemedicine/mindbodyandspirit/music-
therapy

www.cancer.org/treatment/nearingtheendoflife/
index?ssSourceSiteId=null

Cancer Support

---

www.imermanangels.org—"Imerman Angels carefully matches and individually pairs a person touched by cancer (a cancer fighter or survivor) with someone who has fought and survived the same type of cancer (a Mentor Angel). Cancer caregivers (spouses, parents, children and other family and friends of fighters) also receive 1-on-1 connections with other caregivers and survivors. These 1-on-1 relationships inspire hope and offer the chance to ask personal questions and receive support from someone who is uniquely familiar with the experience. The service is absolutely free and helps anyone touched by any type of cancer, at any cancer stage level, at any age, living anywhere in the world." I have been honored to personally meet Jonny, the Founder of Imerman Angels!

www.LiveStrong.org/cancersupport—"At any point in your cancer experience, we provide free, confidential support through education, referrals and counseling services. We can help with: fertility preservation information and assistance, financial, insurance and job concerns, counseling and local resources, and cancer diagnosis and treatment concerns."

www.hopefortwo.org—"Hope for Two…The Pregnant with Cancer Network is a national non-profit organization for women diagnosed with cancer during pregnancy. Our mission is to connect women who are pregnant with cancer with other women who have been pregnant with the same type of cancer. These women are here to lend support, offer hope and share their experiences with one another through phone and e-mail conversation."

www.minniepearl.org — *"Individualized, Just Like You*

"Minnie Pearl offers one-on-one support and guidance to adults (men and women…patient, family member, friend, caretaker, or healthcare professional) impacted by any kind of cancer from the moment of diagnosis. Our support is free of charge and regardless of treatment location. Just as each cancer diagnosis is different, the experience of each person impacted by cancer is different. Because the journey begins at diagnosis and cancer information can be overwhelming, we encourage you to contact us early for education, support and options surrounding your unique needs and circumstances. Our licensed and trained cancer supportive services staff is available for the most reliable and most current

- decision support regarding clinical trials, treatment information, and options
- personalized guidance
- nutrition and side effect management recommendations
- emotional and practical support"

www.cancersupportcommunity.org—"**Our Mission:** To ensure that all people impacted by cancer are empowered by knowledge, strengthened by action, and sustained by community.

"The Cancer Support Community is an international non-profit dedicated to providing support, education and hope to people affected by cancer. As the largest employer of psychosocial oncology mental health professionals in the United States, the organization offers a network of personalized services and education for all people affected by cancer. Its global network brings the highest quality cancer support to the millions of people touched by cancer. To ensure no one has to face cancer alone, these support services are available through a network of professionally led community-based centers, hospitals, community oncology practices and other non-profits, as well as online.

In July 2009, The Wellness Community and Gilda's Club Worldwide joined forces to become the Cancer Support Community. By helping to complete the cancer care plan, the Cancer Support Community continues to optimize patient care by providing essential, but often overlooked, services including support groups, counseling, education and healthy lifestyle programs. Today, the Cancer Support Community provides the highest quality emotional and social support through a network of nearly 50 local affiliates, more than 100 satellite locations and online. To find a community-based center in your area, visit www. cancersupportcommunity.org/FindaCommunity."

www.healingodyssey.org—"Welcome to Healing Odyssey, a nonprofit organization providing recovery and cancer support programs for cancer survivors. Our programs offer the practical tools, skills-building and support needed to cope effectively with the life-altering effects of a cancer diagnosis and treatment. Reconstructing a life that has been devastated by this crisis can be confusing, overwhelming and lonely."

www.cancercare.org — "Cancer*Care* is a national nonprofit, 501 (c)(3) organization that provides free, professional support services to anyone affected by cancer: people with cancer, caregivers, children, loved ones, and the bereaved. Cancer*Care* programs-including counseling and support groups, education, financial assistance and practical help-are provided by professional oncology social workers and are completely free of charge." "All of Cancer*Care*'s services are provided completely free of charge," and they include: counseling, support groups, Connect® Education Workshops, publications, financial help, and other services including community workshops and special events."

Communicating with Others

www.CaringBridge.org—"CaringBridge provides free websites that connect people experiencing a significant health challenge to family and friends, making each health journey easier. CaringBridge is powered by generous donors.

"CaringBridge websites offer a personal and private space to communicate and show support, saving time and emotional energy when health matters most. The websites are easy to create and use. Authors add health updates and photos to share their story while visitors leave messages of love, hope and compassion in the guestbook."

I mentioned previously I built my CaringBridge website within seventy-two hours of confirming my diagnosis. The one additional piece of information I would add is that you can order a book through CaringBridge containing virtually everything from your site. I ordered a book for the first year of my journey called "Year 1!" It is a very nice hardcover book that includes my entire journal, entire guestbook, and photos!

www.mylifeline.org — "Connect. Inspire. Heal. Free, personal websites for cancer patients, survivors and their caregivers. MyLifeLine. org is a 501(c)(3) nonprofit organization that encourages cancer patients and caregivers to create free, customized websites. Our mission is to empower patients to build an online support community of family and friends to foster connection, inspiration, and healing."

Cancer Services

www.lotsahelpinghands.com—"We created Lotsa Helping Hands to answer the question 'what can I do to help?' If you are caring for someone in crisis, or going through one yourself, chances are you have heard this question a lot. And, if you have watched a friend or loved one in need, you have probably asked the same question. Everyone wants to help, but no one knows exactly what to do.

"What is Lotsa Helping Hands? Free, private, web-based communities for organizing friends, family, and colleagues—your 'circles of community'—during times of need. Easily coordinate activities and manage volunteers with our intuitive group calendar.

"Everyone knows what to do and when to do it. Energy is spent helping, not scheduling. Families in crisis are often overwhelmed with many offers of help and phone calls to return. If you are looking for ways to help a friend or loved one, you can create a private community to: organize well-meaning offers of help for meals delivery, rides, and visits, easily communicate and share updates using announcements, message boards, and photos, and safely store vital information."

www.lookgoodfeelbetter.org—"Cancer can rob a woman of her energy, appetite, and strength. But it doesn't have to take away her self-confidence. Look Good…Feel Better is a non-medical, brand-neutral public service program that teaches beauty techniques to cancer patients to help them manage the appearance-related side effects of cancer treatment. Look Good…Feel Better group programs are open to all women with cancer who are undergoing chemotherapy, radiation, or other forms of treatment." I want to emphasize that this site has more than just signing up for a live class. If you cannot get to a class, there are videos, virtual workshops, and a beauty guide with makeup step-by-step, new hair looks, and nail care.

www.livestrong.org/school—"Think your students are too young to face cancer? Think again. With one in three people in the U.S. facing a cancer diagnosis in their lifetime, children in classrooms everywhere are likely to be dealing with cancer right now—with a grandparent, parent, family member, friend or teacher. Research shows that 25 percent of cancer survivors in the U.S. have school-aged children. Also siblings of children with cancer report that the support they receive at school is just as important as the support they receive at home.

"Help your students cope with and learn about cancer. The LIVE**STRONG** at School curriculum offers online lessons for grades K–12 to help you teach your students about cancer in a way that is age-appropriate, inspiring and empowering."

www.fertilehope.org—"Fertile Hope is a national LIVE**STRONG** initiative dedicated to providing reproductive information, support and hope to cancer patients and survivors whose medical treatments present the risk of infertility."

www.musiciansoncall.org—"Musicians On Call brings live and recorded music to the bedsides of patients in healthcare facilities. We believe in the healing power of music. By delivering live, in-room performances to patients undergoing treatment or unable to leave their beds, we add a dose of joy to life in a healthcare facility. Our volunteer artists do more than carry a tune. They deliver it in person.

"The Bedside Performance Program brings live, in-room performances to patients undergoing treatment or unable to leave their hospital beds. It is a program that inspires smiles and thank yous, sing-alongs and tears. And beyond much-appreciated moments of entertainment, these one-on-one interactions between musician and patient have the powerful effect of resurrecting the emotions of joy and happiness that often fade away in healthcare facilities.

"Sometimes a dose of music is just what the doctor ordered. That's why Musicians on Call provides hospitals with CD Pharmacies: complete CD libraries and accompanying disc players for patient use. We currently have CD Pharmacies throughout all 50 states and Washington D.C., as well as Puerto Rico and Ireland."

www.patientadvocate.org—"Our Mission: to provide effective mediation and arbitration services to patients to remove obstacles to healthcare including medical debt crisis, insurance access issues and employment issues for patients with chronic, debilitating and life-threatening illnesses. We assist patients with: medical debt crisis, insurance access issues, and job retention issues."

www.insureustoday.org—"insureUStoday.org is a collaborative effort of healthcare stakeholders to add clarity and take the confusion out of healthcare reform. Our goal is to help improve your understanding of the benefits you will experience as a result of the Patient Protection and Affordable Care Act." This website features a timeline of implementation, interactive blog, helpful resources and informative media articles.

www.tlcdirect.org—"TLC Tender Loving Care is a not-for-profit website and catalog of the American Cancer Society. Our mission is to help women cope during and after cancer treatments by providing wigs and other hair loss products (plus how-to information) as well as mastectomy products."

This is where I personally ordered most of the wigs, hats, and halos (rings of hair) you will see me wearing in the pictures online at www.cancerwithjoybook.com and from my online fashion show on Facebook and CaringBridge.

www.baldisbeautiful.org—"As a fresh-off-the-boat ovarian cancer survivor inspired by my own experience with loss and the many other inner and outer aspects of my journey, I embarked on my *Bald Is Beautiful* mission.

"I want to send a message to women that they can 'flip the script' on the many traumatic aspects of the cancer experience, and embrace every part of their journey with self-love, empowerment, and a deep knowing that their beauty and femininity radiate from within and are not diminished in any way by the effects of having cancer." (Sharon Blynn, Founder of Bald Is Beautiful)

www.cancerandcareers.org—"Cancer and Careers is dedicated to empowering and educating people with cancer to thrive in their workplace by providing expert advice, interactive tools and educational events. Through a comprehensive website, free publications, career coaching, and a series of support groups and educational seminars for employees with cancer and their healthcare providers and coworkers, Cancer and Careers strives to eliminate fear and uncertainty for working people with cancer. Cancerandcareers.org informs more than 180,000 visitors per year, providing essential tools and information for employees with cancer."

www.beingcancer.net—"A Blogging Resource for People Transformed by Cancer: So my intention then for Being Cancer Network was to create a community of people whose lives have been transformed by cancer. The focus for my writing is to stimulate emotion and thought, and to promote sharing of experiences and of what those experiences meant to our gifted and measured lives. Some of this will be history, some stories, other times themes around which we can share our thoughts and feeling. It will become a resource center for a community of cancer bloggers and answer seekers."

www.operationblingfoundation.org—"Operation Bling Foundation's mission is to give sparkling jewels to cancer patients during their hospital stay, bringing them cheer and pleasure. Some women do not feel dressed for the day without their makeup and jewelry; so if bringing bling to women on the oncology floor of hospitals could bring some normalcy and pleasure back to their lives, then that was what Chris was going to do!

"Chris's initial intent was that Operation Bling Foundation's Bling Angels will bring a Bling Gift—for free—to in-patient oncology patients at local hospitals during their hospital stay. She quickly determined that the out-patients during their treatments would also be a perfect place for bling! When a patient is presented with a Bling gift, they will have the choice of a sterling silver cubic zirconium ring, earrings, necklace or bracelet. The Bling gift is presented in a Lucite crystal box enclosed in a white organza pouch. Also enclosed in the pouch is a laminated Bling Card with the foundation's mission statement, an inspirational poem, 'What Cancer Cannot do,' as well as the foundation's logo and contact information."

www.1uponcancer.com/freebies-and-discounts-for-cancer-patients—"Freebies & Discounts for Cancer Patients," with a list including air fare, basic needs, breast prostheses and post-mastectomy bras, camping, classes, dental, gasoline, hats, house cleanings, legal assistance, lodging during treatments, lymphedema alert band, lymphedema sleeves and hand gauntlets, meals, medications/health care, pampering, rent or utilities, retreats, transportation, web-based support community, website, and wigs.

www.happychemo.com—"Discounts, Freebies and Resources for Cancer Patients."

www.cancermatch.com—"CancerMatch is a social network for people fighting cancer." The site also says, "CancerMatch is a powerful cancer survivor networking site. Meet people who are diagnosed with cancer from all over the world. With CancerMatch you can: create a circle of friends who share your diagnosis, or, simply, care about you, build your own network of contacts who share your diagnosis, use built-in communication services to meet or mentor, write your own blog, join a live chat group or person to person chat, post your real life event or attend other members' events, create and lead your own live chat or support group, meet new friends and, maybe, even find a new love."

www.outwithcancer.com —"Out with Cancer is the world's first program for Gay, Lesbian, BI and Trans men and women who are diagnosed with cancer. With Out with Cancer you can: NEW Learn about Clinical Trials…. Search our extensive clinical trial database, create a circle of friends who share your diagnosis, or, simply, care about you, write your own blog, learn from or mentor others dealing with cancer, post photos and profiles, promote your own event or attend other members' events, chat live in online support groups, clubs and one to one sessions, make new friends…OutWithCancer is your place to connect—how is up to you."

Financial Resources

---

www.giveforward.com—"GiveForward is the easiest way to help a loved one in need. GiveForward pages empower friends and family to send love and financial support to patients as they navigate a medical crisis. Create a page today to spread hope and contribute to a loved one's out-of-pocket medical expenses."

www.firstgiving.com—"Be where the giving happens. We help ordinary people raise extraordinary amounts of money for causes they care about. For individual fundraisers, we aim to make it easy, effective, and even fun to raise money online!"

www.aircharitynetwork.org—"Your national charitable aviation network matching people in need with 'free' flights and other travel resources that can provide healing and hope. Every 24 minutes a child or adult in need is being flown through the generous volunteer and donor resources of this charitable aviation network. Air Charity Network™ (ACN) provides access for people in need seeking free air transportation to specialized health care facilities or distant destinations due to family, community or national crisis."

www.hopeflightfoundation.org—"We provide dependable, free air transportation for children who need critical medical treatment for cancer and other life threatening illnesses at facilities far from their homes. We provide a pathway to hope and healing by bridging the gap of distance. Currently we only fly in the states of California, Nevada, and Oregon."

www.cancer.org/treatment/findingandpayingfortreatment/index

Government Websites

www.cancer.gov—"The National Cancer Institute (NCI) is part of the National Institutes of Health (NIH), which is one of 11 agencies that compose the Department of Health and Human Services (HHS). The NCI, established under the National Cancer Institute Act of 1937, is the Federal Government's principal agency for cancer research and training. ... The National Cancer Institute coordinates the National Cancer Program, which conducts and supports research, training, health information dissemination, and other programs with respect to the cause, diagnosis, prevention, and treatment of cancer, rehabilitation from cancer, and the continuing care of cancer patients and the families of cancer patients."

www.cdc.gov/features/womenandcancer—"Centers for Disease Control and Prevention—Your Online Source for Credible Health Information—Every year, cancer claims the lives of more than a quarter of a million women in America. A woman can reduce her cancer risk by adopting a healthy lifestyle and getting the right cancer screening tests for her stage of life."

www.healthcare.gov—"Take health care into your own hands." This website includes the following sections: find insurance options, learn about prevention, compare care quality, understand the law, and information for you (further broken down into: families with children, individuals, people with disabilities, seniors, young adults, and employers).

www.healthcare.gov/law/timeline/index.html—"Understanding the Affordable Care Act Timeline: What's Changing and When." This website has a very nice timeline that shows what changes, when it changes, and gives more information about each change. You can easily read about what has happened and the positive things that are yet to come with healthcare reform.

www.whitehouse.gov/healthreform—"Health reform makes health care more affordable, holds insurers more accountable, expands coverage to all Americans and makes our health system sustainable."

www.pcip.gov—"The Pre-Existing Condition Insurance Plan makes health insurance available to people who have had a problem getting insurance due to a pre-existing condition. The Pre-Existing Condition Insurance Plan: covers a broad range of health benefits, including primary and specialty care, hospital care, and prescription drugs, doesn't charge you a higher premium just because of your medical condition, and doesn't base eligibility on income."

Nutrition

www.cookingwithcancer.org—"Helping those afflicted with cancer to enjoy a better quality of life through good food. Cooking with Cancer is a program designed specifically for cancer care of those persons who are afflicted with cancer, care givers of the patients, and all of those who work in the healthcare industry. The content is recipes researched and tested on patients undergoing chemotherapy and radiation."

www.cancer.org/treatment/survivorshipduringandaftertreatment/nutritionforpeoplewithcancer/index

www.cancer.org/treatment/survivorshipduringandaftertreatment/nutritionforpeoplewithcancer/nutritionforthepersonwithcancer/index

Shops with Cancer Items

www.recoverwithangels.com—"Gift baskets designed for those coping with cancer, other illness, recovery, loss, etc. Our Gift Care Baskets contain carefully selected items designed to comfort, soothe the healing body, mind and soul."

www.cafepress.com/cancerspeaks—"The shop where you can find unique items for the cancer survivor. Great opportunities for you and your loved ones to express the impact cancer has on your lives. Whether you want to promote a little cancer advocacy or a little cancer humor, you can find shirts, cards, mugs and more at the Cancer Speaks store. Great gifts and great friends can come together to lift spirits during difficult times."

Cancer Retreats

www.firstdescents.org—"First Descents offers young adult cancer fighters and survivors (ages 18 to 39) a free week-long outdoor adventure experience designed to enable them to climb, paddle and surf beyond their diagnosis, defy their cancer, reclaim their lives and connect with others doing the same" I personally attended a First Descents rock-climbing camp in late September 2010 in Boulder, Colorado. It was a wonderful experience to meet and get to know other young adults who live different places, had been through a diverse variety of cancer treatments, and all came together in a very supportive environment.

www.castingforrecovery.org—"We provide an opportunity for women whose lives have been profoundly affected by the disease to gather in a natural setting and learn the sport of fly fishing. Just as importantly, the retreats offer an opportunity to meet new friends, network, exchange information, and have fun.

"Our weekend retreats incorporate counseling, educational services, and the trained facilitators that staff each retreat, including a psycho-social therapist, a health care professional (e.g., physical therapist, nurse), as well as fly-fishing instructors and river helpers.

"While the fundraising burden of offering healing retreats at no cost to participants and asking volunteers to run state programs is enormous, Casting for Recovery has inspired the generous and loyal support of donors large and small, and continues to believe in its mission of providing women with powerful tools for healing at no expense to them."

www.reelrecovery.org—"The mission of Reel Recovery is to help men in the cancer recovery process by introducing them to the healing powers of the sport of fly-fishing, while providing a safe, supportive environment to explore their personal experiences of cancer with others who share their stories."

www.bluebirdmi.org—"Through the unique experience of weekend programs, Bluebird Cancer Retreats participants have a very special opportunity for listening and learning, not only about their disease, but insights from others like themselves who live with cancer. Participants will find time to reflect, share, and learn about coping with cancer while participating in a variety of educational, recreational, and social activities. Bluebird's weekend retreats are held on the shores of Lake Michigan at the Camp Geneva Conference Center. Located just 5 miles north of Holland, Michigan, Camp Geneva's beautiful facilities and breathtaking natural surroundings provide the ideal setting in which to experience respite and renewal for those on the cancer journey."

www.bcrecovery.org—"All retreats are designed by breast cancer survivors for breast cancer survivors. Breast Cancer Recovery embraces all women with breast cancer including all faiths, ages, races, sexual orientations and financial resources. Women in all stages are welcome to attend—from the newly diagnosed to women many years in remission. Women ages 20–71 have attended a retreat."

www.cocai.org—"The Children's Oncology Camping Association International (COCA-I) includes over 65 camps for children and young adults across the U.S., Canada, and the world, most of which are free or have only nominal application fees. The mission of COCA-I is to promote and strengthen the international community of camps for children with cancer and their families through networking, advocacy, and education.

For a complete listing of COCA-I camps, alphabetized by camp name and by state/province, visit www.cocai.org or call 706-799-1002."

www.campkesem.org—"Camp Kesem is a college student run summer camp for kids with a parent who has (or has had) cancer. Our one-week sleep away camps are a chance for kids 6–13 to have a fun-filled week and just be kids." Some programs also accommodate teens 14-16.

Young Adults

www.planetcancer.org—"LIVE**STRONG** recognizes that young adults with cancer slip into a lonely no-man's land. Too old for the instant community of a children's hospital, they still don't fit in with the over-50 community that overwhelmingly populates adult cancer wards. Because young adults with cancer are a relatively small group, the difficulty of finding peer support is increased exponentially, forcing many to deal in isolation with issues specific to this age and stage of life: dating with cancer, disclosure to a potential employer, long-term insurance issues, moving back home, loss of fertility, or having to quit school or a newly launched career. Planet Cancer exists so that no young adult will have to endure such isolation again.

"Online Community—The My Planet social network is the world's largest online community of young adults who have been affected by cancer. It's a place where members find and communicate with other young adults around the world about what's on their minds—from death or fertility issues to dumb things people say.

"Weekend retreats—Our weekend retreat program brings together young adults for recreation and personal exploration with their peers, helping them forge connections that will sustain them as they move on with their lives, in or out of treatment. We currently offer programs for: 18–25 year olds, 25–40 year olds, and young couples under 40 facing cancer together."

www.ulmanfund.org—"A leading voice in the young adult cancer movement, we are working at a grassroots level to support, educate, connect and empower young adult cancer survivors. Since inception in 1997, we have been working tirelessly at both the community level and with our national partners to raise awareness of the young adult cancer issue and ensure all young adults and families impacted by cancer have a voice and the resources necessary to thrive. Our work over the years and to present day is guided by both our mission, vision and values and priorities and goals set forth within our strategic plan."

One of the many things I found at their website is a college scholarship program.

www.vitaloptions.org—"Vital Options International is a not-for-profit cancer communications, support, and advocacy organization with a mission, to facilitate a global cancer dialogue.

"Founded in 1983 by Selma Schimmel when she was diagnosed at 28 with breast cancer, Vital Options was the first psychosocial and advocacy organization for young adults with cancer. In 1996 with the launch of the Group Room cancer talk radio show, Vital Options evolved into a cancer communications organization for people of all ages. Vital Options is noted for its pioneering and innovative approaches in using cutting edge technology to advocate and communicate about cancer through a variety of audio and video formats. Additional projects include The CancerNewsMinute®, CancerTalk℠, CancerTours™, The Professor & The Survivor®, Advocacy in Action®, and National Young Adult Cancer Awareness Week®.

"In 2000, Vital Options became an international organization and today works with the patient advocacy and professional oncology community throughout the United States and Europe. Its programs enable patients and their loved ones to interact directly with leading worldwide oncology opinion leaders regarding the latest advances in cancer treatment, research, advocacy, and public policy issues. All Vital Options services are offered without charge."

www.stupidcancer.com—"I'm Too Young for This! 70,000 Americans between 15–40 are diagnosed with cancer each year. That's one every eight minutes. It's also seven times more than all childhood cancers combined. This is not OK! We exist to ensure that these young adults are made aware of—and given access to—our global support community and the wealth of age-appropriate resources that they are entitled to so they can get busy living."

Caregivers, Family, and Friends

www.caregivers4cancer.org—"Unless you have a medical degree or background, chances are you don't know how to care for a cancer patient. As the wife of a cancer patient, I was thrust into this role and didn't have a clue what to do, but I learned quickly, although not always easily. This is the scariest roller coaster ride of your life!

"If you are: dealing with a loved one or friend who has cancer, trying to get through the maze of healthcare, need a resource to help you stay the course, overwhelmed but don't want your loved one to know, you've come to the right place."

www.caregiverslibrary.org—"The National Caregivers Library was created by FamilyCare America, Inc. and is one of the largest single sources of information and tools for caregivers and seniors in the country. It makes its resources available to caregivers for free through alliances with professionals, businesses and other organizations who serve seniors and their caregivers with a variety of products and services.

"The library consists of hundreds of useful articles, forms, checklists and links to topic-specific external resources. It is organized into logical categories that address the key needs of caregivers and their loved ones. The library also includes an entire section for employers."

www.youngcancerspouses.com—"Our mission is to bring together young spouses of adults with cancer to share information, support, and experiences.

"The needs of young spouses of cancer patients often go unrecognized and unappreciated. The emotional and logistical issues a young spouse of a cancer patient faces are vastly different from spouses of older cancer patients that dominated oncology units and support groups. General family support groups are likewise inadequate at addressing the needs of a young cancer spouse. At YoungCancerSpouses, we seek to provide a source of practical information gained from our experience as young cancer spouses. We also strive to bring together other young cancer spouses to share ideas, lend support, and validate their wide range of feelings and emotions so they can find comfort in an understanding community."

www.circusofcancer.org—"A how-to site to help you step right up when your friend has breast cancer." I enjoyed the *How to Help Your Friend* link which gives tips in the following areas: "upon first hearing the news, boosting her spirits, helping her family, supporting chemo, talking to your friend, for her husband or partner, and great sites for small gifts."

Contributor Websites

www.JanHasak.com—Jan is a contributor of one of the stories in chapter three. Her website has an amazing resources list you should check out, including: breast cancer general information, hospital and government cancer information, cancer blogroll, breast cancer treatment decisions, managing side effects of chemo and herceptin, beauty issues, young breast cancer survivors, breast cancer advocacy and fundraising groups, general cancer advocacy groups, breast reconstruction (or not), general cancer information, cancer clinical trials, support groups, retreats, discussion boards on cancer and related issues, lymphedema books, lymphedema general information, lymphedema products (not all inclusive, just some major ones), lymphedema blogroll, support groups specifically for lymphedema, cancer caregiving, fitness for breast cancer survivors, general health, vitamins and herbal supplements/alternative and integrative medicine, grieving, cleaning assistance, legal assistance, financial assistance, and health insurance affordability.

www.thereislifeafterbreastcancer.com—This is the website of contributor Hayley Townley, and it includes survivor stories, a blog, a place you can share your story, and a resources section.

www.elainejesmer.com—The website of contributor Elaine Jesmer. Links to www.chemotalk.com and a sign-up for the Chemotalk newsletter.

www.facingbreastcancer.com—The website of contributor Lois Hjelmstad. There is a wonderful tab with articles here!

www.thanksforthememoirs.com— This is the website of contributor Marie Rowe. "Telling your story to a Personal Historian and having those remembrances presented in a book with special photos, is a lasting and priceless gift for your family and friends to enjoy and cherish. It's your imprint on the world...your voice, your spirit, your soul and your heart. I believe that be recalling life experiences and accomplishments, enhances our appreciation of who we are today. Capture the stories of your lifetime with Thanks for the Memoirs!"

www.JoyHuber.com—My website, and a place where you can read about my LIVE "Cancer with Joy" program I bring into hospitals and cancer treatment centers. I also speak to many support and survivor groups and at conferences, events, etc. You can read about all my programs at www.JoyHuber.com/programs and book me to speak by going to www.JoyHuber.com/contact and filling out the form completely or by e-mailing details of your request to bookings@cancerwithjoy.com.

Make sure you sign-up at www.cancerwithjoybook.com and become a member. You receive two months FREE with your purchase of this book! At this site I will send you spaced out reminders of these resources (because I know this list can be a little overwhelming, but, as you scan the descriptions, you will see which ones best meet your immediate needs). Members will also receive bonus sites as new resources come to my attention. If you want to share a useful site not found in this list for consideration, e-mail it to resources@cancerwithjoybook.com. At the membership site, I will also send out updated links if any of these become non-functional. To report a link that is not working for you, e-mail brokenresources@cancerwithjoybook.com.

Now, find out how to access the big bonus! All of this is just the beginning.

Claim Your Bonus

I have mentioned many times throughout this resource that this is just the beginning of many ways I am here with you to help you handle "Cancer with Joy." There is a FREE two-month trial membership in the "Cancer with Joy" community waiting for you at the website at the bottom of this page. As a member of this community, you will interact with and receive:

1. Pictures of my personal journey from diagnosis through treatment

2. Video from my personal journey from diagnosis through treatment

3. Music (including songs co-written by me)—"Bright Side Effects" and "Live Before I Die"

4. The *latest* cancer news

5. Recipes

6. **MORE** stories from other cancer patients and survivors

7. **MORE** resources and updates on where to find resources mentioned in chapter nine if the links change

8. The "Cancer with Joy" store where you can order T-shirts and more!

9. Updates from me on my personal story

10. Information on events (find out where I'm appearing!)

AND MORE! (I'm saving some Exciting *Special Surprises* NOT listed here for Members ONLY!)

Special Discounts Too but ONLY for "Cancer with Joy" Community Members!

This special gift from me is **valued at over $60** and is yours just for purchasing this book!

Join Today

www.CancerwithJoyBook.com

Recipes

I share this website in the resources chapter as well. www.cookingwithcancer.org has a recipes tab and I wanted to share ½ dozen recipes with you. What I enjoyed about this site is how all the recipes are searchable. If you are looking for a recipe that could be therapeutic for something particular you are experiencing, you can try these below. I selected recipes that state they are specifically for: mouth inflammation, constipation, stimulating taste, dehydration, digestion, and diarrhea.

Melon Soup with Lime Sorbet

Cuisine: Fruit Course: Soup Therapeutic: Mouth Inflammation

Ingredients:
- 1 Melon, skinned and diced (about 1 Pound)
- Orange Juice orange only 1 each
- Lemon Juice Lemon only 1 each
- Sparkling water 2 cans 12 fluid ounces
- Orange zest grated 1 Tbsp (table spoon)
- Lemon zest grated 1 Tbsp (table spoon)
- Cornstarch 1/2 Tbsp
- Habanero pepper powder for seasoning (to taste)
- Salt or Sugar for seasoning (to taste)

Steps:

Garnish: lime sorbet

1. Puree melon and orange juice in the blender and place in the refrigerator.

2. Mix lemon juice, sparkling water and zests. Bring to boil.

3. Stir in the cornstarch to lemon juice mixture for thickening and chill in the refrigerator.

4. Stir melon puree and adjust seasoning. If salty appeals season with salt or if sweet appeals season with sugar. Habanero pepper is needed to intensify the flavor.

5. Serve cold in a deep plate and garnish with lime sorbet in a ball in the center.

Sorbet can be obtained in the frozen food section at the local grocery store. This is to stimulate the sensation of color for the patient and the temperature will add extra sensation of coolness.

Plantain Croquettes

Cuisine: Fruit Course: Appetizer Therapeutic: Constipation

Ingredients:

Plantain is a relative to the banana and has a significant effect on intestinal function, providing the body with help on days of hyper or diminished bowel function.

- Plantain, medium sized, ripe 2
- Black bean paste (refried black beans) 4 ounces (oz)
- Hot pepper of choice (recommend coban pepper) to taste
- Sugar to taste

Steps:

1. Peel the plantain and puree to form a soft but firm dough (add mashed potatoes if needed)
2. Flavor with sugar and pepper.
3. Use a medium sized skillet with a dash of olive oil to heat refried black bean paste. Allow to cool. Place a tablespoon full of black bean paste in the middle of a plantain patty and mold in to a croquette or a ball. Fry the croquettes on a sauté pan to golden color. Sprinkle with sugar and enjoy.

Black Bean Puree (refried) with Blanco Cheese and Tomato Sauce

Cuisine: Mexican Course: Main Course Therapeutic: Stimulating Taste

Ingredients:

Black beans are the backbone to the diet for many Latin countries including Guatemala, Cuba and Brazil. The combination of cheese and gently spiced tomato sauce enhances the taste, while providing gentle stimulation to the large bowel function.

- Refried black bean (easily obtained from the grocery store) 1 can
- Onion, finely chopped ½
- Olive oil 1 teaspoon
- Blanco cheese 1
- Ripe tomato, seeded, peeled and diced 1
- Jalapeno pepper powder pinch
- Salt and pepper to taste

Steps:

For the beans:

1. In a frying pan with oil, blanch the onions.
2. Add black bean and mix well on medium heat.
3. Frequently stir to avoid crusting, until the dough has a paste consistency.
4. Pass to a plate and refrigerate.

For the tomato sauce:

1. In a frying pan place same amount of oil and onion until blanched.
2. Add tomato, well mixed and cook. Add a pinch of jalapeno pepper powder to taste.

3. Putting together: Cut the cheese and black bean paste in matching triangles 2 inches in length, ½ inch wide. Place then standing and opposing; gently fill the bottom of the plate with tomato sauce and garnish with fresh parsley leaves.

Grilled Watermelon, Melon and Cheese in Tamarindo

Cuisine: Fruit Course: Main Course Therapeutic: Dehydration

Ingredients:
This recipe is rich on water and sugars. It assists in rehydration and calorie intake during dehydration. The meaty flesh of the fruit stimulates the gums.

- Watermelon, seeded and cut in large rectangles 1
- Melon, seeded and cut in large rectangles 1 each
- Queso fresco, cut in matching rectangles 1

For the Tamarindo sauce:
- Tamarindo fruit ½ pound (2 cups)
- Sugar to taste
- Hot pepper to taste

Steps:

1. Place the Tamarindo fruit, skinless on water and gentle simmer for one hour.
2. Allow to cool and separate the seeds. Blend the mixture and reduce on low heat.
3. When at sauce point (coats the back of the spoon). Add sugar to taste. Sprinkle over the watermelon, melon and cheese.

Anise Ice Cream with Honey Vodka Caramel

Cuisine: Egg product Course: Dessert Therapeutic: Digestion

Ingredients:

Anise and its seeds have been around for a long time. This recipe will help colic (spasmic pains) not only during premenstrual syndrome (PMS) but also infantile colic syndrome. In addition, this recipe includes alcohol/vodka acting as a significant tranquilizer to help stimulate appetite.

For the ice cream:
- Anise extract 1 oz. by volume
- Lactate free milk 16 ounces (1 pint)
- Sugar to taste

For the cone:
- Vodka 2 ounces
- Honey 4 ounces

Steps:

For Ice Cream:
1. In a sauce pan, place the ingredients together and bring gently to a boil. Please be careful as it will get hot.
2. Place the mixture in an ice cream maker and following the recommendation by the manufacturer, spin until double in size.
3. Place in the freezer until ready to use.

For Basket:
1. In a sauce pan place the ingredients together and bring gently to boil. Please be careful as it will get hot. As becomes thick or reaches an internal temperature of 220 degrees Fahrenheit; gently pour on a glass or metal mold to become a basket. Allow to cool. For serving: Garnish with anise flowers or mint as available.

Guava Cupcakes

Cuisine: Fruit Course: Dessert Therapeutic: Diarrhea

Ingredients:

Guava is a tropical tree. Over centuries the fruit bark and leaves have been used as a home remedy for gastrointestinal ailments, in particular, diarrhea.

- Guava fruit, clean 4
- Cinnamon sticks 2
- Water 2 cups
- Instant Coffee 3 teaspoons
- Brown Sugar 2 ounces
- Queso fresco, cut into 1x1x1 inch squares 12
- Cupcake liners 12

Steps:

1. Place the guava, cinnamon sticks and water together in a sauce pan. Bring to boil and simmer for 5 minutes.

2. Separate the fruit and cool in the refrigerator. Then slice into ½ inch slices and remove seeds.

3. Combine liquid from sauce pan with the instant coffee and brown sugar and boil together until caramelized.

4. Cool in the refrigerator.

5. Heat oven to 350 degrees Fahrenheit.

6. Place cupcakes liner on flat pan, and place one queso fresco square inside each liner.

7. Warm in oven until gently melted (approx. 5 minutes). Place slice of guava in to the melted cheese and then let cool. At the serving time add a teaspoon full of coffee caramel and gently sprinkle with habanero pepper dust.

A Special Discount
Only for Readers of
"Cancer with Joy" on *"You Go Girl"* (My First Book)

My first book for women in business on dealing with difficult people is part of a system that can be accessed immediately at <u>www.ManageDifficultPeopleNow.com</u>. EVERY woman knows 'difficult people' unfortunately, and needs effective tips for thriving around them so she can feel better immediately!

This system includes six bonuses (audio, insiders' & bonus reports, AND music!) and is only $47.

Since you have purchased my second book, "Cancer with Joy" I want to give you a deep discount on my first book

"You Go Girl: A Woman's Guide on How to THRIVE Around Difficult People."

Go to: <u>www.ManageDifficultPeopleNow.com/specialoffer</u>

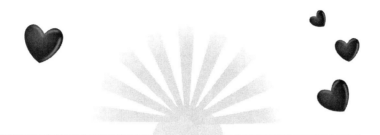

About the Author

Joy Huber is a stage four young adult cancer survivor and the founder of "Cancer with Joy." She is an award-winning international presenter, individual coach, and songwriter.

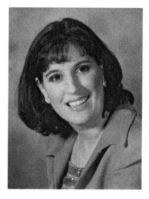

Joy Huber

Joy helps the newly diagnosed and those on their support team learn how to transform fear into happiness with resources, support, and en'courage'ment. She wrote "Cancer with Joy" to be the essential resource for the newly diagnosed providing helpful and highly valuable information that saves precious time, energy, and money. Joy is an inspiration, and her humor and positive energy ignites others to transform their experience with cancer from negative to "Cancer with Joy."

Joy's clients have included large companies and small business, the government, colleges, associations, and hospitals. Her "Cancer with Joy" presentation is highly sought-after by cancer treatment centers, hospitals, support groups, and survivor rallies. Book "Cancer with Joy" at www. joyhuber.com/contact.

References

Canfield, Jack with Janet Switzer. 2005. *The Success Principles: How to Get from Where You Are to Where You Want to Be.* New York: HarperCollins.

Last Holiday. 1996. Paramount Pictures.

nutrition. Dictionary.com. *The American Heritage® Science Dictionary.* Houghton Mifflin Company. http://dictionary.reference.com/browse/nutrition (accessed: July 05, 2011).

Swindoll, Charles. 1982. "Attitude."

Davis, Richard and Joy Huber. 2009. "Live Before I Die" (lyrics).

Green, Marv and Steve Diamond. 2009. "Consider Me Gone" (lyrics).

Huber, Joy and Bob Paterno. 2010. "Bright Side Effects" (lyrics).

Overstreet, Paul and Don Schlitz. 1987. "Forever and Ever Amen" (lyrics).

"What Cancer Cannot Do." (n.d.).

BUY A SHARE OF THE FUTURE IN YOUR COMMUNITY

These certificates make great holiday, graduation and birthday gifts that can be personalized with the recipient's name. The cost of one S.H.A.R.E. or one square foot is $54.17. The personalized certificate is suitable for framing and will state the number of shares purchased and the amount of each share, as well as the recipient's name. The home that you participate in "building" will last for many years and will continue to grow in value.

Here is a sample SHARE certificate:

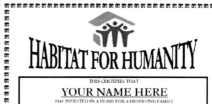

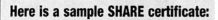

HABITAT FOR HUMANITY

THIS CERTIFIES THAT
YOUR NAME HERE
HAS INVESTED IN A HOME FOR A DESERVING FAMILY

1985-2010
TWENTY-FIVE YEARS OF BUILDING FUTURES
IN OUR COMMUNITY ONE HOME AT A TIME

1200 SQUARE FOOT HOUSE @ $65,000 = $54.17 PER SQUARE FOOT
This certificate represents a tax deductible donation. It has no cash value.

YES, I WOULD LIKE TO HELP!

*I support the work that Habitat for Humanity does and I want to be part of the excitement! As a donor, I will receive periodic updates on your construction activities but, more importantly, I know my gift will help a family in our community realize the dream of homeownership. **I would like to SHARE in your efforts against substandard housing in my community!** (Please print below)*

PLEASE SEND ME _____ SHARES at $54.17 EACH = $ $_____

In Honor Of: _____

Occasion: (Circle One)   HOLIDAY   BIRTHDAY   ANNIVERSARY

OTHER: _____

Address of Recipient: _____

Gift From: _____ *Donor Address:* _____

Donor Email: _____

I AM ENCLOSING A CHECK FOR $ $_____ PAYABLE TO HABITAT FOR HUMANITY **OR** PLEASE CHARGE MY VISA OR MASTERCARD *(CIRCLE ONE)*

Card Number _____ Expiration Date: _____

Name as it appears on Credit Card _____ Charge Amount $ _____

Signature _____

Billing Address _____

Telephone # Day _____ Eve _____

PLEASE NOTE: Your contribution is tax-deductible to the fullest extent allowed by law.
Habitat for Humanity • P.O. Box 1443 • Newport News, VA 23601 • 757-596-5553
www.HelpHabitatforHumanity.org

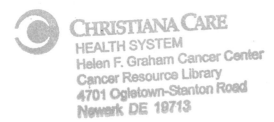
CPSIA information can be obtained at www.ICGtesting.com
Printed in the USA
BVOW020154170212

283080BV00002B/6/P